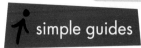

simple guides

Thyroid disorders

Dr Eleanor Bull
Dr John Reckless

Thyroid disorders
First published – April 2006

Published by
CSF Medical Communications Ltd
1 Bankside, Lodge Road, Long Hanborough
Oxfordshire, OX29 8LJ, UK
T +44 (0)1993 885370 F +44 (0)1993 881868
enquiries@bestmedicine.com
www.bestmedicine.com

We are always interested in hearing from anyone
who has anything to add to our Simple Guides.
Please send your comments to *editor@csfmedical.com*.

Author Dr Eleanor Bull
Managing Editor Dr Eleanor Bull
Medical Editor Dr John Reckless
Science Editor Dr Scott Chambers
Production Editor Emma Catherall
Layout Jamie McCansh and Julie Smith
Operations Manager Julia Savory
Publisher Stephen I'Anson

© CSF Medical Communications Ltd 2006

All rights reserved

ISBN-10: 1-905466-09-9
ISBN-13: 978-190546-609-2

The contents of this *Simple Guide* should not be treated as a substitute for
the medical advice of your own doctor or any other healthcare professional.
You are strongly urged to consult your doctor before taking, stopping or
changing any of the products or lifestyle recommendations referred to in this
book or any other medication that has been prescribed or recommended by
your doctor. Whilst every effort has been made to ensure the accuracy of the
information at the date of publication, CSF Medical Communications Ltd and
The Patients Association accept no responsibility for any errors or omissions or
for any consequences arising from anything included in or excluded from this
Simple Guide nor for the contents of any external internet site or other
information source listed and do not endorse any commercial products or
services mentioned.

Printed in Italy.

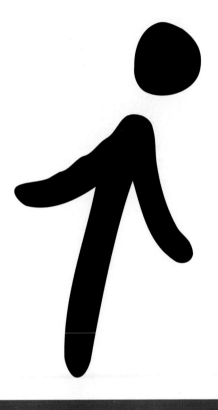

FOREWORD

TRISHA MACNAIR
Doctor and BBC Health Journalist

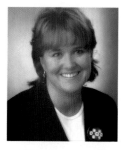 Getting involved in managing your own medical condition – or helping those you love or care for to manage theirs – is a vital step towards keeping as healthy as possible. Whilst doctors, nurses and the rest of your healthcare team can help you with expert advice and guidance, nobody knows your body, your symptoms and what is right for *you* as well as you do.

There is no long-term (chronic) medical condition or illness that I can think of where the person concerned has absolutely no influence at all on their situation. The way you choose to live your life, from the food you eat to the exercise you take, will impact upon your disease, your well-being and how able you are to cope. You are in charge!

Being involved in making choices about your treatment helps you to feel in control of your problems, and makes sure you get the help that you really need. Research clearly shows that when people living with a chronic illness take an active role in looking after themselves, they can bring about significant improvements in their illness and vastly improve the quality of life they enjoy. Of course, there may be occasions when you feel particularly unwell and it all seems out of your control. Yet most of the time there are plenty of things that you can do in order to reduce the negative effects that your condition can have on your life. This way you feel as good as possible and may even be able to alter the course of your condition.

So how do you gain the confidence and skills to take an active part in managing your condition, communicate with health professionals and work through sometimes worrying and emotive issues? The answer is to become better informed. Reading about your problem, talking to others who have been through similar experiences and hearing what the experts have to say will all help to build up your understanding and help you to take an active role in your own health care.

Simple Guides provide an invaluable source of help, giving you the facts that you need in order to understand the key issues and discuss them with your doctors and other professionals involved in your care. The information is presented in an accessible way but without neglecting the important details. Produced independently and under the guidance of medical experts *Thyroid disorders* is an evidence-based, balanced and up-to-date review that I hope you will find enables you to play an active part in the successful management of your condition.

What happens normally?

WHAT HAPPENS NORMALLY?

The thyroid gland helps to regulate the growth of our bodies and the rate of our metabolism (the processes that include the conversion of food that we eat into energy our bodies can use). In other words, it controls the speed at which our bodies work.

SMALL BUT VITAL

Although our thyroid gland is tiny – weighing less than 20 grams (the mass of a squash ball) – we would soon miss it if it wasn't there. The thyroid is an endocrine gland, which means that it manufactures hormones, which are important chemical messengers that circulate around the body in the bloodstream and govern the way in which our bodies work.

Situated in your neck, just beneath your voice box (or Adam's apple), the thyroid is made up of two halves (the left and right lobes). Some people think that the shape of the thyroid resembles a butterfly's wings. The two lobes lie on either side of your wind pipe and are linked together by a narrow portion of thyroid tissue called the isthmus.

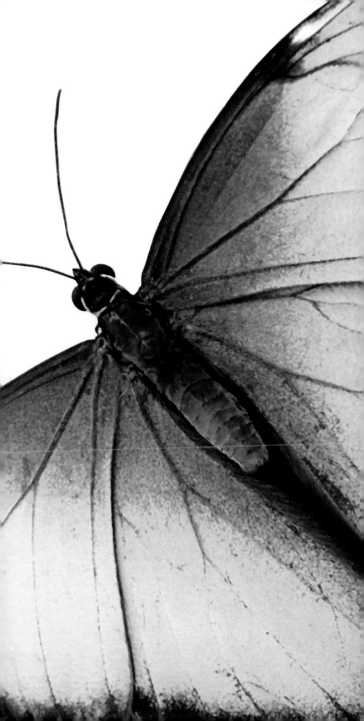

WHAT DOES THE THYROID DO?

The thyroid is responsible for the manufacture of two important hormones:

■ thyroxine (also known as T4)

■ triiodothyronine (pronounced *try-eye-odo-thigh-ron-neen*; also known as T3).

The levels of thyroid hormones in our bodies usually remain fairly constant. Thyroid hormones have two general functions.

■ **Controlling our metabolism**
Both thyroid hormones can increase the speed at which the body processes carbohydrates, fats and proteins. They can also act on the heart, liver, kidney and muscle to increase the consumption of oxygen and production of heat by the body.

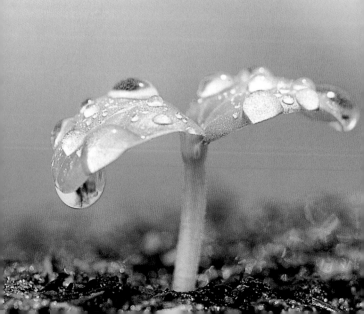

■ **Controlling our growth and development**

Thyroid hormones can directly regulate the growth of the cells of our body, as well as influencing the production of growth hormone by the pituitary gland (a hormone gland that hangs on a stalk at the base of the brain). They are therefore essential for normal physical growth and mental development, especially during childhood.

WHAT ARE THE PARATHYROID GLANDS?

The parathyroid glands, of which we have four, are adjacent to our thyroid gland. The parathyroid glands are not related to the thyroid except by their position. These glands produce parathyroid hormone (PTH) which regulates the concentration of calcium and phosphorus in the blood. Calcium is essential for healthy bones as well as for general well-being so it is important that the amount of calcium circulating through our bodies is carefully controlled.

5

IODINE AND THE THYROID GLAND

Most of the iodine found in the body is located in the thyroid gland. Iodine is an essential raw material for the manufacture of thyroid hormones. Triiodothyronine contains three atoms of iodine and is often called T3. Thyroxine contains four atoms of iodine and for this reason is often called T4. To exert its effects within the body, T4 must be converted to T3 inside the body (by removal of a single iodine atom).

In the UK, getting enough iodine is not usually a problem because it is found in a variety of foods, including fruit and vegetables, meat (especially liver), enriched cereals, seafood and seaweed. Remember though, that consuming too much iodine can aggravate existing thyroid conditions.

An atom is the smallest component of an element (e.g. iodine) that retains the chemical properties of that element. The word 'iodine' comes from the Greek word 'iodes', meaning 'violet colour'.

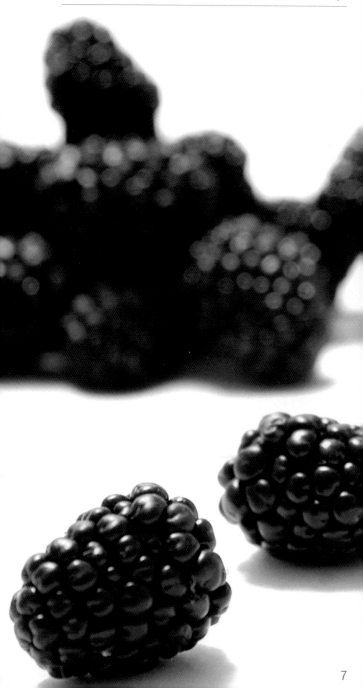

WHAT CONTROLS THE THYROID?

The activity of the thyroid gland is carefully regulated by the pituitary gland and the hypothalamus. The pituitary is a hormone gland that hangs on a stalk at the base of the brain and the hypothalamus is located above the pituitary and forms part of the brain itself. These work as a team (known as the hypothalamic–pituitary–thyroid axis).

By working in concert, the hypothalamus, pituitary gland and the thyroid gland control levels of thyroid hormones in our bloodstream very tightly.

■ If there is too much T4 and T3 in the blood then the hypothalamus will sense this and will respond by ceasing production of thyrotropin-releasing hormone (TRH) which thereby slows down the production of thyroid hormones. This process of control is called negative feedback.

■ If the pituitary gland cannot detect very much T4 and T3 in the bloodstream then it will make more thyroid-stimulating hormone (TSH) which will indirectly lead to more thyroid hormones being produced.

The whole system is a bit like a boiler and a thermostat. The pituitary gland senses and controls the levels of thyroid hormones in your bloodstream, just as the thermostat in your house senses and controls the temperature. When it becomes too cold, the thermostat senses the temperature and fires up the boiler (the thyroid). When the heat rises to the set temperature, the thermostat senses this and the boiler cuts out.

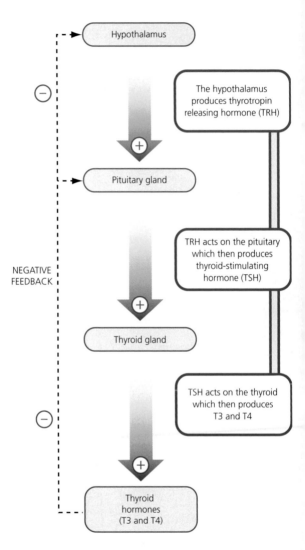

THE PRODUCTION OF THYROID HORMONES IS CONTROLLED BY A SPECIFIC CHAIN OF EVENTS.

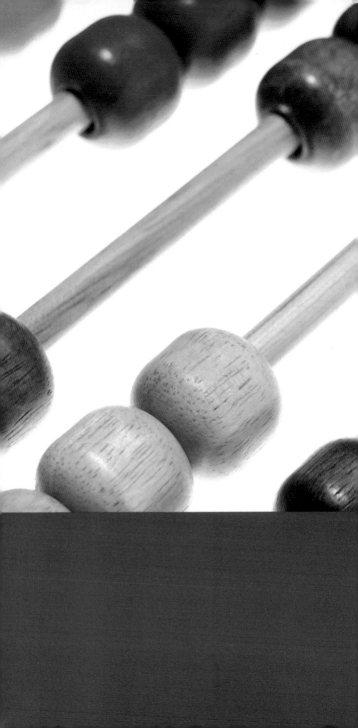

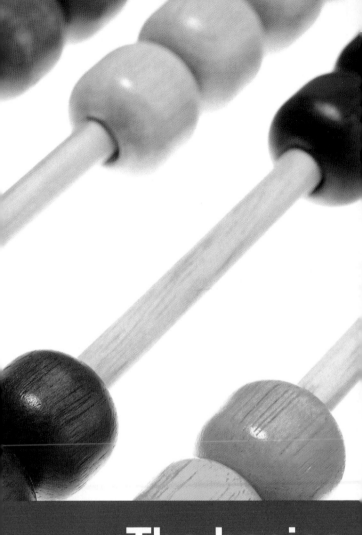

The basics

THYROID DISORDERS – THE BASICS

If something goes wrong with your thyroid, you may not notice immediately because symptoms can come on gradually and vary enormously from person to person. Whilst thyroid disorders cannot usually be prevented – they can be managed effectively given the right treatment.

Under normal circumstances, the thyroid gland functions smoothly and we are blissfully unaware of it and the important job it is doing for us. Medically, this state is known as euthyroidism. However, when the thyroid gland either produces too little or too much of the thyroid hormones, the balance is disrupted and symptoms emerge. There are two major types of thyroid disorder.

1. **Hypothyroidism** – occurs when the thyroid gland releases too few thyroid hormones into the bloodstream. Too little hormone tends to slow down the body's functions.

2. **Hyperthyroidism** – occurs when the thyroid gland becomes overactive and releases too many thyroid hormones into the bloodstream. Too much hormone can make the body's functions speed up.

So, in essence, thyroid disorders are all about an imbalance in thyroid hormones. But what happens exactly? It may help to consider the thermostat and boiler analogy described in *What happens normally?* (page 8). Consider the thyroid

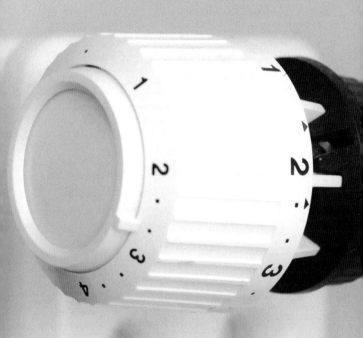

gland as a boiler (controlling the temperature and metabolic rate of the body) and the pituitary gland as the thermostat that controls the temperature of the 'boiler'. Thyroid disorders come about when the 'thermostat' (the pituitary gland) cannot read the temperature accurately or when the 'boiler' (the thyroid) fails to respond appropriately to the thermostat.

Hypo means 'under' or 'below normal'
Hyper mean 'over' or 'above normal'.

SYMPTOMS

The symptoms of a thyroid disorder vary hugely from person to person, ranging from barely noticeable to completely debilitating. Some people develop very severe symptoms even though their thyroid function only differs modestly from normal. The reverse is also true – some people may experience only mild symptoms but their thyroid function may be rather abnormal. It all depends on the individual. Some thyroid disorders may go undetected for many months because the symptoms can easily be confused with other conditions like the menopause or stress.

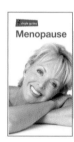

For more information see
Menopause

Symptoms of hypothyroidism (an underactive thyroid)

There are many different symptoms of hypothyroidism, and shown below are a few of the most common ones. As you will see, some of these symptoms (like tiredness) are relatively common complaints and suffering from them may often not mean that you have a problem with your thyroid. The more unusual symptoms (like a lump in the front of the neck) are a more reliable indicator of thyroid disease:

- tiredness; always in need of sleep

- increased awareness of the cold

- dry and thickened skin and hair

- puffy face and bags under the eyes

- heavier, prolonged periods

- unexplained weight gain

- depression, lack of concentration

- raised blood pressure, slow heart beat

- swelling at the front of the neck

- pins and needles in the fingers and hands

- flaking, splitting nails

- hair loss, especially the outer third of the eyebrow.

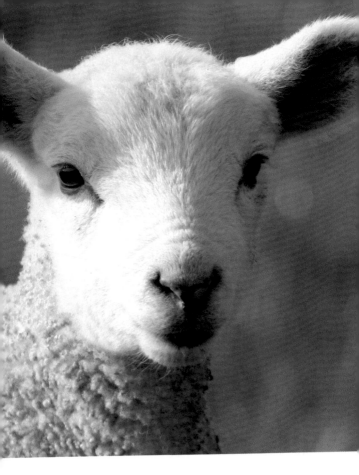

Symptoms of hyperthyroidism (an overactive thyroid)

There are many different symptoms of hyperthyroidism, and shown below are a few of the most common ones:

- disturbed sleep
- feeling hot, increased sweating
- hair loss
- brittle nails
- periods are lighter or absent

- palpitations

- nervousness, anxiety

- hyperactive behaviour (may be particularly noticeable in children)

- unexplained weight loss

- protruding eyeballs or vision problems

- swelling at the front of the neck

- rapid growth in children.

Thyroid nodules and cysts

A thyroid nodule is a (usually small) lump in an otherwise normal thyroid gland. If one nodule forms, then this is called solitary adenoma. If more than one forms, this is called multinodular goitre. Thyroid nodules are very common and do not usually cause any symptoms as such, although you may sometimes feel a lump in your throat or may be able to see a lump in your neck. Very rarely, tests can reveal that these nodules are malignant, but some are simply cysts (a mass containing a fluid or a semisolid substance).

GOITRE

If the thyroid becomes sufficiently enlarged it can cause swelling which (depending on its size) may start to protrude visibly from the neck. Your doctor may be able to feel a lump when he or she examines you. This is called a goitre and may be the most obvious sign of a thyroid disorder.

If the thyroid gets very large it can very occasionally press on the gullet or windpipe. Whether the thyroid is of normal or enlarged size does not determine whether its overall hormone production is normal, low or high. Euthyroidism, hypothyroidism or hyperthyroidism can all be associated with a goitre. There are different types of goitre.

■ **Diffuse smooth goitre**
Here the entire thyroid gland is larger than normal. If the goitre is very big then you may experience difficulties swallowing or even breathing properly.

■ **Nodular goitre**
Here, there are single or multiple small lumps within the thyroid (single or multinodular), which may have arisen as a result of a cyst, a benign tumour (an adenoma) or rarely a malignant cancerous tumour.

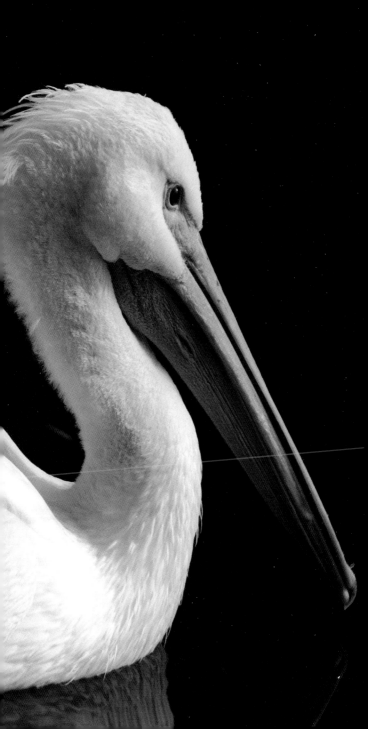

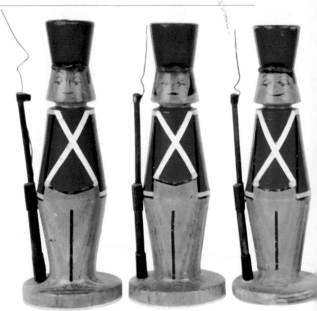

AUTOIMMUNE THYROID DISEASE

Autoimmune disease is brought on when the body's immune system mistakes healthy cells, organs, or tissues in the body for foreign invaders and starts attacking them. There are two major types of autoimmune thyroid disease – **Hashimoto's disease** (leading to hypothyroidism) and **Graves' disease** (leading to hyperthyroidism). Whilst the symptoms of these two conditions are different, they are both caused by a malfunctioning immune system and hence are termed 'autoimmune diseases'.

Our immune systems protect us from foreign invaders (like bacteria and viruses) by destroying them with specially tailored substances called antibodies. Under normal circumstances our immune system helps to protect us against infection and without it we would not survive. However, if

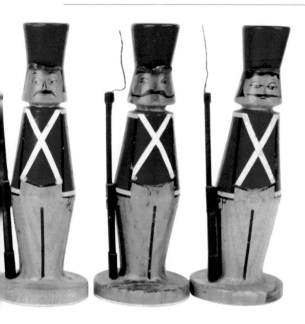

you have an autoimmune disease, then your body starts to make antibodies that are directed against particular parts of the body itself, thereby destroying particular groups of cells or tissues within the body.

If you have an autoimmune thyroid disease, your body has mistaken your thyroid as a 'foreign body' and attacks it. This damages the gland so that it doesn't function properly and releases abnormal amounts of thyroid hormones. Rheumatoid arthritis is another type of autoimmune disease.

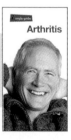

For more information see
Arthritis

WHAT CAUSES HYPOTHYROIDISM?

■ **Autoimmune disease.** Hashimoto's disease (also called Hashimoto's thyroiditis) is the most common example of autoimmune thyroid disease. This arises when the body's immune system mistakenly attacks the thyroid gland.

■ **Radioiodine therapy** for the treatment of hyperthyroidism (see page 36).

■ **Surgical removal of the thyroid gland** for the treatment of hyperthyroidism, thyroid cancer or removal of a very large goitre that is interfering with your swallowing or breathing (see page 36).

■ **Inflammation of the thyroid gland** (thyroiditis).

■ **Post-partum thyroiditis.** This is a temporary underactivity (or sometimes overactivity leading to hyperthyroidism)

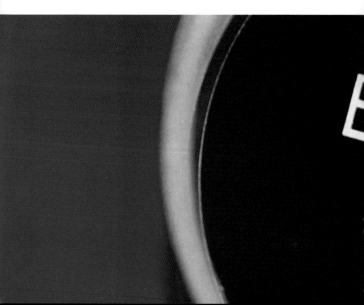

of the thyroid gland in some women following childbirth.

- **Certain types of medication.** Drugs like lithium (used to treat certain psychiatric illnesses) and amiodarone (used to correct abnormal heart rhythms [arrhythmias]) can cause thyroid problems.

- **Congenital hypothyroidism.** A condition some babies are born with. Occurs when the thyroid gland fails to develop properly in the womb. Blood tests performed in the days following birth can pick up this condition (as well as other congenital conditions).

- **Malfunction of or damage to the hypothalamus or pituitary gland**, both of which control that activity of the thyroid gland.

- **Lack of iodine in the diet.** This is exceedingly rare in the UK these days, but not everyone in the world has a diet that is rich in iodine.

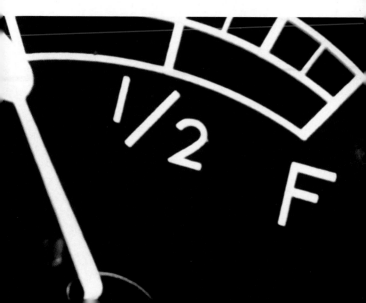

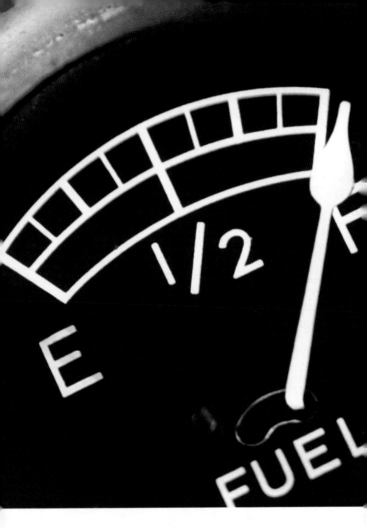

WHAT CAUSES HYPERTHYROIDISM?

■ **Graves' disease.** The most common cause of hyperthyroidism in the UK. Arises when the body's immune system mistakenly attacks the thyroid gland.

■ **Nodules** (small lumps) in the thyroid gland (nodular thyroid disease) can sometimes affect thyroid function.

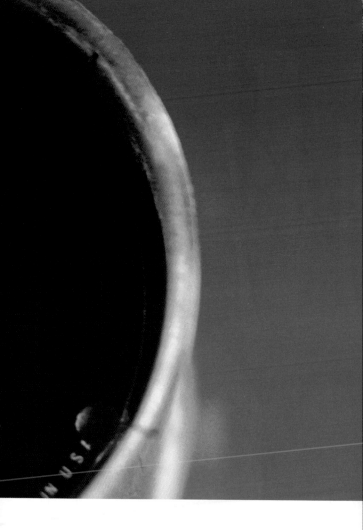

■ **Excessive doses of thyroid hormone replacement therapy** (e.g. T3 and T4 [or thyroxine]). These hormone tablets are used to treat hypothyroidism.

■ **Too much iodine in the diet.** This is rare in the UK.

THE COMPLICATIONS OF THYROID DISORDERS

Having a thyroid disorder can sometimes make you more likely to develop other diseases or can worsen existing medical conditions. If levels of thyroid hormones become too high (as a result of hyperthyroidism) palpitations and a heart condition known as atrial fibrillation can result. Here the electrical impulses within the heart become erratic and if left untreated, this can bring out serious heart conditions like angina or precipitate heart failure.

Hyperthyroidism can also make you more likely to develop osteoporosis. Hypothyroidism (low levels of thyroid hormones) can sometimes increase the levels of cholesterol circulating in the bloodstream which is a risk factor for coronary heart disease.

Some of the diseases sometimes associated with autoimmune thyroid disease are listed in the adjacent table.

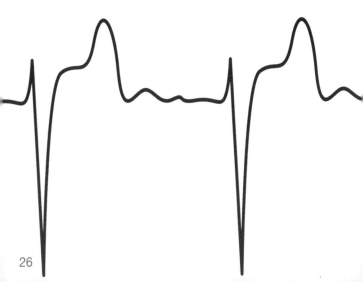

COMPLICATIONS SOMETIMES ASSOCIATED WITH AUTOIMMUNE THYROID DISEASE

Addison's disease	Occurs when the adrenal glands, sitting above the kidneys, fail to function properly. Symptoms include weakness and low blood pressure.
Alopecia	Partial or complete hair loss.
Type 1 diabetes mellitus	Occurs when the body is unable to produce the hormone insulin and hence properly regulate sugar (glucose) levels in the blood. Symptoms include hunger, thirst, excessive urination, dehydration and weight loss.
Eye disease	Graves' ophthalmopathy (see overleaf).
Myasthenia gravis	A muscle disease that can affect the muscles of the eye, face, lips, tongue, throat or neck. Can eventually affect more than one of these regions. Occurs when the body's immune system fights the muscles.
Pernicious anaemia	A type of anaemia (lack of red blood cells) caused by a deficiency in the proteins that handle vitamin B12 in the body.
Vitiligo	Occurs when the immune system attacks the pigment-producing cells within the skin. This results in prominent white patches and some areas of increased pigmentation on the skin surface.

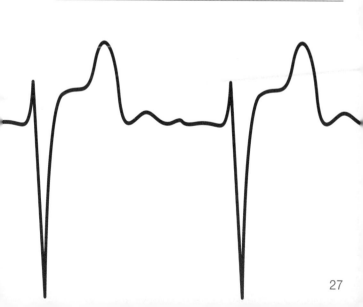

Graves' ophthalmopathy

A fair proportion (but not all) people with Graves' disease develop a form of eye disease as a consequence of the underlying hormonal imbalance. This is known as Graves' ophthalmopathy. In some cases eye symptoms may develop before the hyperthyroidism. In other cases, they may develop some years after an overactive thyroid has been corrected with treatment. If you have Graves' disease and you smoke, you are more likely to develop severe Graves' ophthalmopathy. Most people with Graves'

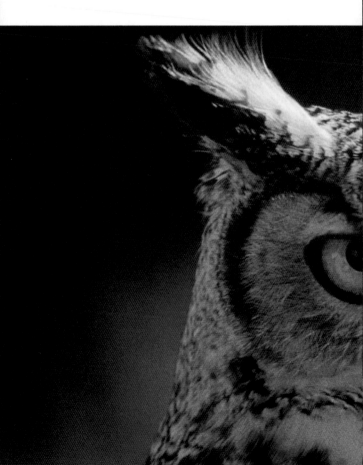

ophthalmopathy will experience only minor and temporary changes in their eye appearances and/or vision, but some people can suffer from:

- puffiness of the eye lids

- a staring look

- a swelling of the eye muscle that pushes the eyes forwards in their sockets

- double vision or even loss of vision

- pain.

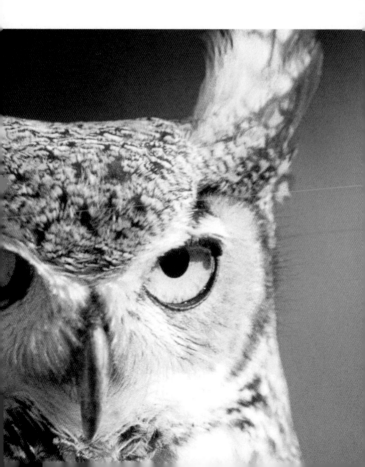

DIAGNOSING THYROID DISORDERS

Your symptoms can develop over a matter of weeks or it may take many months before you notice them, which may prompt you to go and see your doctor. If you suspect that you may have a thyroid disorder, it is important that you seek medical advice. However, the chances are that your doctor will have detected your thyroid disorder during a routine check-up or when you go to see them about a seemingly unrelated complaint.

Your doctor will be able to get a good idea about the activity of your thyroid gland by:

- listening to you describe your symptoms

- asking you about your medical history

- asking you about the medical history of your family

- looking for specific physical signs (like goitre, a fast pulse, sweating or eye symptoms)

- examining your neck for signs of swelling

- their overall impression of you as you walk into the consultation room.

The symptoms experienced by people with thyroid disorders vary so much that a blood test is the only way to confirm whether or not you have one. Your doctor will only arrange a blood test if they suspect you have a thyroid disorder and not as a matter of course.

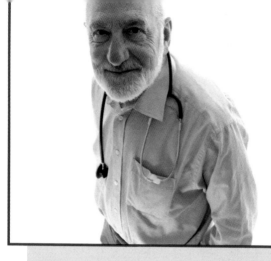

GP

As a GP, I will probably be your first port of call. My role is to recognise and diagnose your thyroid disorder and to start the management process. You may come to me because you are concerned about the symptoms you have been experiencing, or I may pick up on your thyroid problem during a routine consultation for a seemingly unrelated complaint.

In order to make an accurate diagnosis, I will ask you about your symptoms and your medical history, and do a physical examination. If I suspect a thyroid disorder, I will take a sample of blood to be analysed in a laboratory. The outcome of this test will govern exactly how your thyroid complaint is managed from here on in. If you have hypothyroidism, I will usually be able to manage you in my surgery.

This can mean offering advice and reassurance, recommending lifestyle changes and prescribing medication if appropriate. If hyperthyroidism is diagnosed, then it is routine for me to refer you to see a specialist, usually in a hospital. Even though I may not be managing you, you should feel free to come and talk to me about your thyroid disorder.

Thyroid function

Carrying out a blood test will determine the levels of various thyroid hormones that you have circulating in your bloodstream. The concentration of thyroid-stimulating hormone (TSH) in particular can give important clues as to how well your thyroid gland is working because it reflects your body's view of the thyroid hormone situation. TSH is the hormone released by the pituitary gland that tells the thyroid gland what to do, like the thermostat controlling the boiler.

If the levels of thyroid hormones in the blood become too low then the pituitary gland responds by producing more TSH in an attempt to boost thyroid hormone production (or *vice versa*). This explains why levels of TSH are high in a person who has an underactive thyroid.

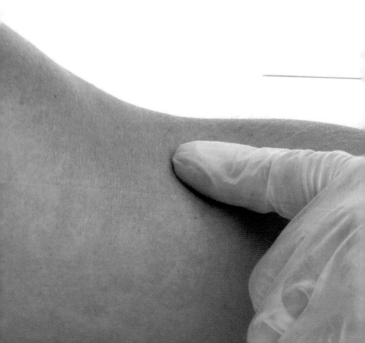

Thyroid disorder	Thyroid hormone		
	TSH	Free T3 (T3)	Free T4 (T4)
Hypothyroidism	High	Low	Low
Subclinical hypothyroidism	Raised	(Low) Normal	(Low) Normal
Hyperthyroidism	Low	High	High
Subclinical hyperthyroidism	Low	(High) Normal	(High) Normal

Guide normal values*: TSH 0.3–5.5 mu/L; fT3 3.9–6.8 pmol/L; fT4 12–22 pmol/L.

*Values will vary somewhat from laboratory to laboratory (see *Managing thyroid disorders page 68*).

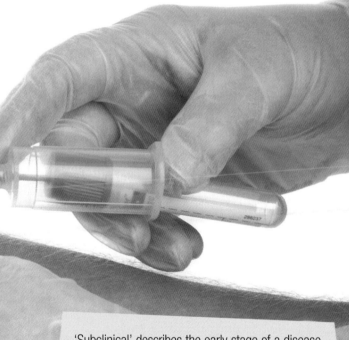

'Subclinical' describes the early stage of a disease or condition, before symptoms become noticeable.

MANAGING THYROID DISORDERS

The course of treatment you will be recommended largely depends on what type of thyroid disorder you have been diagnosed with. If you have hypothyroidism then you will usually be managed by your GP at your local surgery and you will probably need to take thyroid hormone replacement therapy for the rest of your life.

Rest assured that this should not affect your daily routine. If you have been diagnosed with hyperthyroidism then it is usual practice to refer you to a specialist doctor, called an endocrinologist, who specialises in thyroid problems.

Treating goitre

If your goitre is not malignant, is relatively small or is not causing you any symptoms, then your specialist may feel that it is best left as it is. If your goitre is large and unsightly (or is causing pressure symptoms in the neck) then your doctor may recommend that you undergo surgery to have it removed. Before deciding on a course of treatment, your doctor will check the levels of thyroid hormones in your bloodstream to see if you have underlying hypo- or hyperthyroidism, and may test the cells inside the swelling to see whether they are benign or malignant.

Treating hypothyroidism

You will usually be offered **thyroid hormone replacement therapy.**

- Levothyroxine sodium (thyroxine) and liothyronine sodium (triiodothyronine) are the two synthetic thyroid hormones currently available in the UK. These thyroid hormones are identical to the body's own hormone. Your body cannot tell whether the thyroxine has come from your thyroid, or from tablets, or from a mixture of both.

- Your thyroid function will gradually return to normal (over a number of weeks) but you will usually have to keep taking thyroid hormone replacement therapy for the rest of your life.

- You will have a blood test 2–3 months after starting thyroid hormone replacement therapy to check that your TSH levels have returned to normal, and every year thereafter to check that they have stayed normal.

- Over the years, you may find that the dose of thyroid hormone you need to take goes up. The initial replacement dose may be a partial dose, but over subsequent months or years you may need to go up to a full dose.

Treating hyperthyroidism

You will usually be offered treatment with antithyroid medication, radioiodine treatment or surgery, or a combination of these.

■ **Antithyroid medications** are carbimazole (Neo-Mercazole®) and propylthiouracil. They work by slowing down the manufacture of thyroid hormones by the thyroid gland. Most people notice that their symptoms subside after 2–5 weeks of treatment. Once they have subsided, treatment is usually continued for a period of 18 months.

■ **Radioiodine treatment** involves swallowing radioactive iodine (as a capsule or less often, a drink). It is automatically taken up by the thyroid gland as a raw material for the manufacture of thyroid hormones. The radioiodine concentrates in the thyroid gland and destroys some of the thyroid tissue, thereby slowing the manufacture of thyroid hormones.

■ A **thyroidectomy** is the partial or total removal of the thyroid gland by surgery. If you have your thyroid gland removed completely then you will have to take thyroid hormone replacement therapy for the rest of your life.

If they are managed effectively, thyroid disorders need not disrupt your day-to-day way of living. It is important that you take responsibility for yourself and make sure you take your medication as directed and attend regular check-ups with your doctor or specialist. Becoming better informed about your thyroid disorder may help you to deal with it more effectively – reading this book is a great place to start!

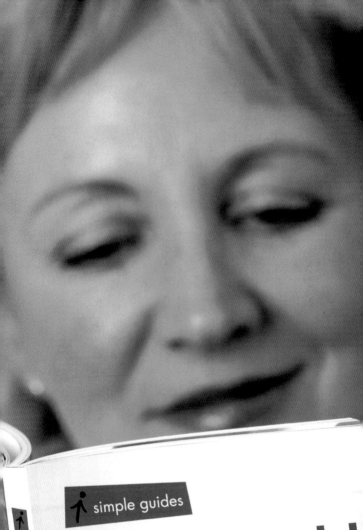

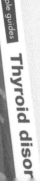

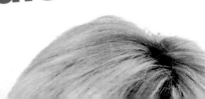

simple guides

Thyroid
disorders

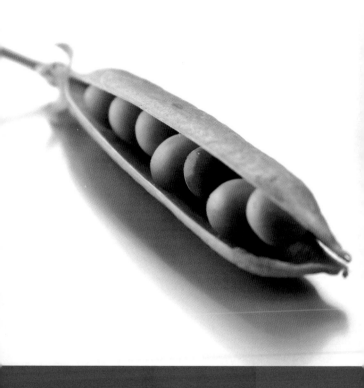

Why me?

WHY ME?

Around one person in every twenty will experience a thyroid disorder at some point in their lives. Hashimoto's thyroiditis and Graves' disease are amongst the most common causes of hypo- and hyperthyroidism, respectively.

HOW COMMON ARE THYROID DISORDERS?

If you, or someone you know, have recently been diagnosed with a thyroid disorder, you are by no means alone. Thyroid disorders are very common indeed. Estimates suggest that one in every twenty people is affected by a thyroid disorder at some point in their lives. Because the signs and symptoms can vary so much, it is sometimes difficult to recognise a thyroid disorder for what it actually is. It is only when symptoms don't

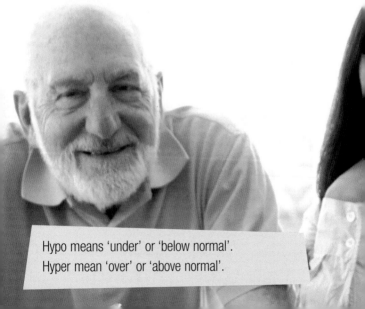

Hypo means 'under' or 'below normal'.
Hyper mean 'over' or 'above normal'.

improve or become more severe that people tend to seek medical advice. This may mean that the prevalence of thyroid problems is actually higher than the estimates suggest.

In the UK, the most common cause of hypothyroidism is Hashimoto's disease whilst Graves' disease is the most common cause of hyperthyroidism. As we described in *The basics* (page 20), both of these diseases are types of autoimmune disease and occur when the body produces an antibody that mistakenly attacks the thyroid gland. Autoimmune disease tends to run in families. Generally speaking, thyroid disorders are more common in women than men, especially during our 20s and 30s.

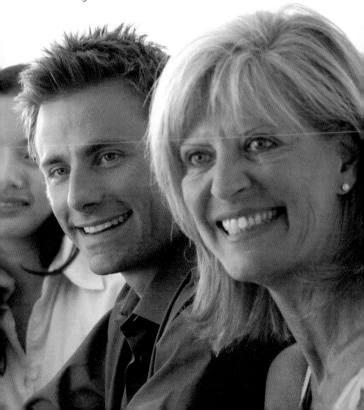

As we mentioned earlier, thyroid nodules are very common in both men and women. Whilst most of these are benign (and some will be cysts), a low percentage turn out to be malignant thyroid nodules and must be managed accordingly (see *The treatment of thyroid cancer,* page 112).

THYROID CANCER

Thyroid cancer is extremely rare and represents only 1% of all types of cancer. Each year, there are about 1,400 new cases in the UK. Thyroid cancer can occur at any age and is slightly more common in women than in men. Most importantly, it can be very successfully treated if it is caught early enough (see *The treatment of thyroid cancer,* page 112).

NUCLEAR FALLOUT AND RADIOTHERAPY

Many Russian children caught up in the Chernobyl nuclear disaster in 1986 went on to develop thyroid cancer as a result of the extremely high levels of radiation they were exposed to in the immediate aftermath of the incident.

Furthermore, it may seem paradoxical but the 'radiotherapy' used in the past to treat cancer and some other types of disease, may actually cause cancer itself. Evidence shows that people who have had radiotherapy to their neck have an increased risk of thyroid cancer later in life (often after 10–30 years).

The risk is particularly great if this treatment took place during childhood. It is therefore very important that you are not exposed to any more radiation than is absolutely necessary. Rest assured that the radioiodine therapy you may receive if you have been diagnosed with hyperthyroidism will not cause cancer.

INHERITING THYROID CANCER

It is possible (although very rare) that you may have inherited a susceptibility to developing thyroid cancer. Some people with a condition known as Multiple Endocrine Neoplasia type 2 (MEN 2) carry an abnormal gene that can make them more likely to develop medullary thyroid cancer (cancer that affects the cells in the thyroid that produce calcitonin, a hormone that helps to control the levels of calcium in the bloodstream) at some stage in their life. There are two types of MEN (MEN 1 and MEN 2), both are rare and both are inherited.

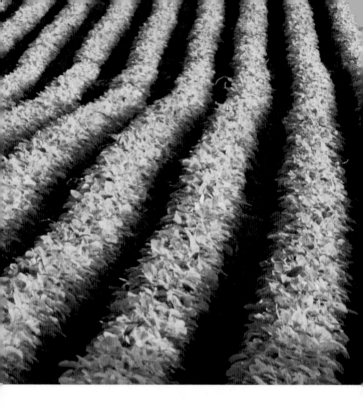

LOCATION, LOCATION, LOCATION

You may be surprised to learn that the health of your thyroid gland can depend on where you live. This is because some regions of the world are iodine deficient, that is to say, the concentration of iodine in the soil (and hence in the foods that are grown in that soil) is very low. This can have important health implications. In the worst cases, a severe and prolonged lack of iodine in the diet can lead to irreversible mental retardation in children.

Worldwide, some degree of iodine deficiency affects over 1,575 million people (almost 30% of the world's population) across 110 countries. Yet, it is easily preventable with iodised salt (salt that is fortified with iodine).

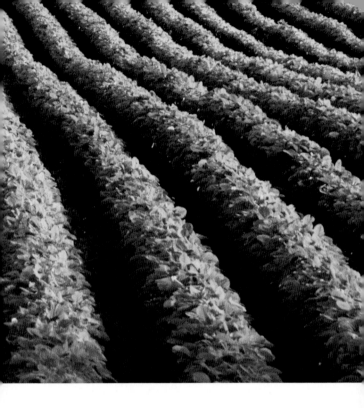

The World Health Organization is working hard to give iodine deficient areas better access to this cheap commodity.

Closer to home, iodine deficiency is thankfully no longer a problem. However, only a couple of decades ago there were pockets of iodine-deficient areas, most notably in Derbyshire, where the soil and rock lacks iodine. People living in Derbyshire were more likely to develop goitres than those people living in iodine-rich areas. So much so that 'Derbyshire neck' became a recognised medical term. In this age of the supermarket – no single region is dependent on locally grown food for its dietary intake of iodine and Derbyshire neck is now rarely seen.

HOW DID I END UP WITH A THYROID DISORDER?

When some people are first diagnosed with a thyroid disorder, they initially hold themselves responsible and question whether it was something they did or didn't do that caused it. This is extremely unlikely. Thyroid disorders are usually down to factors beyond our control, such as the following.

■ **Age**

Although thyroid problems can affect anyone at any age, hypothyroidism tends to be more common in older people. This may be because the thyroid shrinks as we age, which slowly reduces the amount of thyroid hormones available to the body.

■ **Sex**

Women are more likely to be affected by a thyroid disorder than men. For example, it has been estimated that women are ten-times more likely to develop hyperthyroidism than men. There is also considerable overlap in the symptoms of thyroid disease and the menopause and sometimes the two are confused, which can complicate diagnosis.

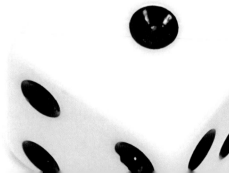

■ Family history

Autoimmune thyroid disorders like Hashimoto's thyroiditis and Graves' disease tend to run in families.

■ Medical history

If you or a close blood relative suffer from another autoimmune disease, like type 1 diabetes mellitus, vitiligo or Addison's disease, you are more at risk of developing a thyroid condition (see *The basics* page 27).

■ Medication

Some types of medication can affect the normal functioning of the thyroid gland. These include, amongst others, lithium (for some psychiatric disorders) and amiodarone (for abnormal heart rhythms; 'cardiac arrhythmias').

■ Previous surgery

You may have been treated in the past for goitre, hyperthyroidism or thyroid cancer that involved the complete or partial removal of the thyroid gland itself. This may have caused you to go on to develop hypothyroidism.

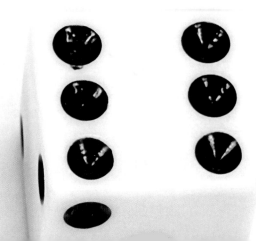

THYROID DISORDERS IN CHILDREN

The thyroid gland has a very important role to play in newborn babies and young children, not just because of its effects on metabolism but also because of the important role it plays in growth and development.

In some babies, the thyroid gland may not have developed properly or does not function as it should (some babies are even born without a thyroid gland, although this is very unusual). This is called congenital hypothyroidism, and affects one in every 3,500 to 4,000 babies born in the UK each year. In the UK, all newborn babies are screened for a thyroid disorder when they are a few days old so any abnormalities are picked up early and treated accordingly. Your doctor or midwife will take a blood sample by pricking your baby's heel (also known as the Guthrie test; named after the American scientist Robert Guthrie, who first designed the test in 1963).

Some children (who have normal thyroid function at birth), may go on to develop a failing thyroid in later life (during child- or adulthood). If the thyroid fails in childhood then you may notice that your child:

- tires easily
- has a small appetite but puts on weight easily
- is often constipated
- has difficulty concentrating at school
- has a poor memory
- is short for their age or shows slow growth.

The symptoms of hyperthyroidism tend to emerge at a later age in children. Affected children may:

- appear restless
- show disruptive behaviour
- have difficulty concentrating at school
- have a very large appetite but fail to put on any weight
- be particularly tall for their age.

Again, childhood hyperthyroidism is diagnosed by a blood test and is easily corrected, with much the same treatment as is used in adults (see *Managing thyroid disorders* page 68).

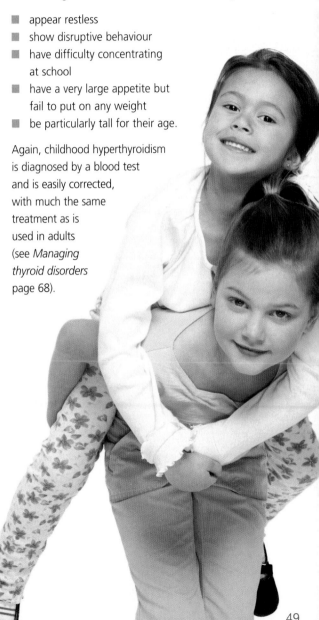

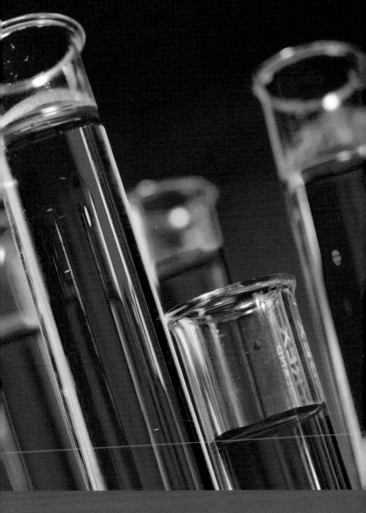

Simple
science

SIMPLE SCIENCE

Learning how your thyroid should function normally and what goes wrong when you have a thyroid disorder can help you to understand your thyroid condition and may make it easier to live with.

As we have already seen, our thyroid gland regulates our metabolism and controls the rate at which we use energy. When our thyroid doesn't work as it should then a number of things can occur:

- **hypothyroidism** – the thyroid is underproductive

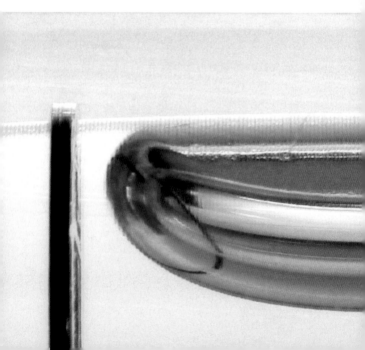

- **hyperthyroidism** – the thyroid goes into overdrive

- **goitre** – the thyroid is enlarged

- **thyroid nodules** – single or multiple lumps develop in the thyroid

- **thyroid cancer**.

But why should this happen in the first place? This section will concentrate on the first two points, hypo- and hyperthyroidism. In the UK the most common cause of these disorders relates to abnormalities in the immune system, the body's natural form of defence against disease or infection.

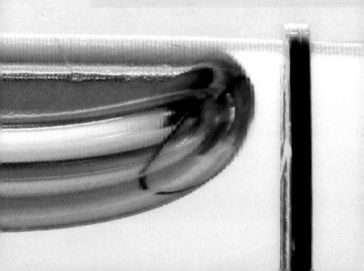

MANAGING THYROID DISORDERS IS ABOUT REBALANCING THE LEVELS OF THYROID HORMONES.

A CASE OF MISTAKEN IDENTITY

Some of the most common thyroid disorders
(e.g. Hashimoto's thyroiditis and Graves' disease)
can be traced back to a malfunction in the
immune system, wherein the body produces
antibodies that attack the cells of the thyroid
gland because it mistakes it for a foreign invader.
We touched on this autoimmunity briefly in
The basics (page 20).

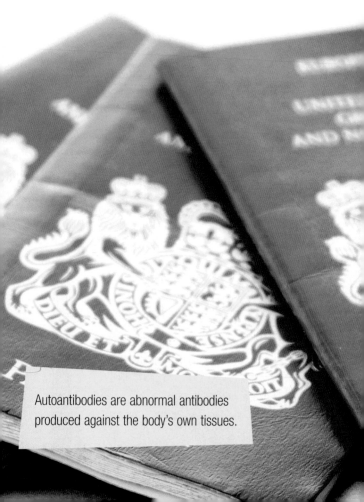

Autoantibodies are abnormal antibodies
produced against the body's own tissues.

The antibodies that your body produces in these circumstances are called autoantibodies. Some autoantibodies are destructive and (together with other types of immune cell) kill off the thyroid cells, causing hypothyroidism (e.g. Hashimoto's thyroiditis). Other antibodies stimulate the thyroid cells to produce too many thyroid hormones, causing hyperthyroidism (e.g. Graves' disease).

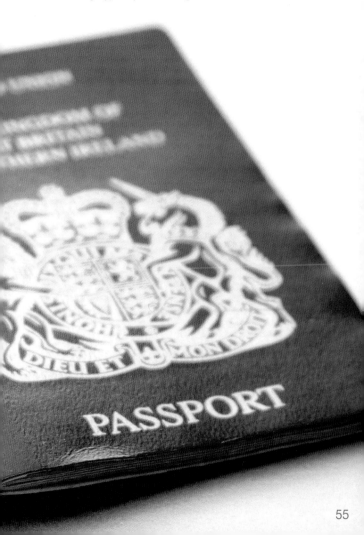

THE IMMUNE RESPONSE

So what are antibodies and what do they do exactly? Antibodies are made by white blood cells called B-lymphocytes. They can be thought of as Y-shaped structures, with a special region at the tip that recognises and attaches to a specific foreign substance, called an antigen. This is known as the antigen binding site. Once it has attached to the antibody, the antigen is neutralised.

Every antigen has a specific and unique antibody. For example, if the body becomes infected with a particular type of flu virus (an antigen) it will generate a specific anti-flu antibody against it. This antibody will simply not recognise anything other than the flu virus it was made to target. Some antibodies (like those made against diseases like chicken pox or measles) can protect us for a lifetime, whereas others (like those made against the flu virus) are temporary, and are rendered useless when the virus evolves, or changes.

Our blood is made up of three types of cell:

■ White blood cells
■ Red blood cells (which help to carry oxygen around our bodies)
■ Platelets (which help to form blood clots).

White blood cells are a key part of the body's defence mechanism against infection.

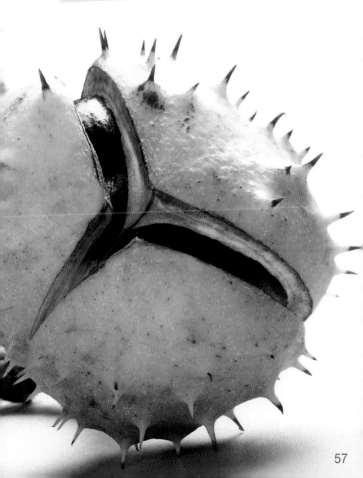

Once the antibody has been released by the B-lymphocyte in response to the presence of an antigen, it then recognises and attaches itself to the antigen and a whole host of reactions are triggered. Collectively, these reactions are known as the immune response. The purpose of the immune response is to neutralise the antigen and eliminate (or delete) it from the body. It is the antibody that kick-starts the immune response.

Of course, if the immune response is triggered inappropriately, perfectly healthy and harmless cells and tissues can be damaged. This is what happens when autoantibodies are made in people with autoimmune thyroid diseases, although it should be borne in mind that a percentage of people who have autoantibodies do not have (and never develop) an autoimmune disease.

In Hashimoto's disease, the antibody and the immune lymphocytes may attack the thyroid, causing it to work less effectively than normal. In Graves' disease, the antibody attaches itself to the thyroid gland and stimulates the release of thyroid-stimulating hormone (TSH), causing the thyroid to become overactive.

As we have seen, Graves' disease is also associated with a number of eye problems like disturbed vision and protruding eyeballs (see *The basics* page 28). These occur when the autoimmune response affects not only the thyroid gland but spills over to the cells behind the eyeball and makes them swell up, forcing the eyeball outwards. It is unclear why some people with Graves' disease develop thyroid eye disease and others don't, but scientists are investigating why this happens.

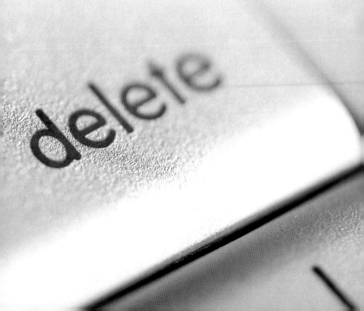

HOW DO WE TREAT AUTOIMMUNE THYROID DISEASE?

The more we understand autoimmune thyroid diseases, the easier they will be to treat and even prevent. At the moment, there are some gaps in what we know. For example, what makes some people more likely than others to develop autoimmune disease or what makes the immune system suddenly decide to produce autoantibodies?

For now, all we can do is treat the symptoms of autoimmune thyroid diseases, and use a combination of drugs, surgery or radiation to restore the balance of thyroid hormones to what it should be (see *Managing thyroid disorders* page 95).

Treating thyroid disorders is about rebalancing levels of thyroid hormones...

Hypothyroidism – Synthetic thyroid hormones boost the body's levels of thyroid hormones.

Hyperthyroidism – Antithyroid drugs, radioiodine and/or surgery block the production of thyroid hormones.

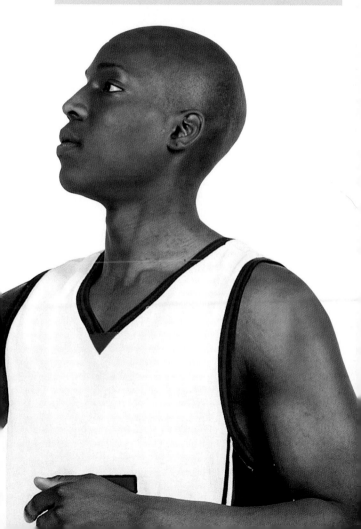

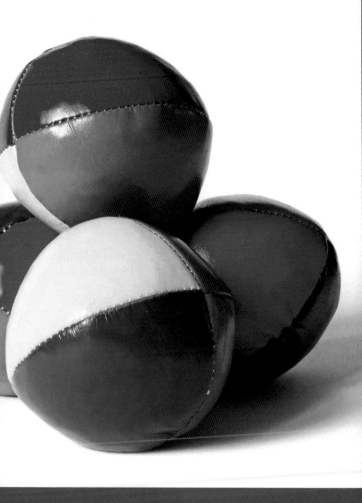

Managing
thyroid
disorders

MANAGING THYROID DISORDERS

Although managing a thyroid disorder can be a lifelong commitment, it need not become a life sentence. By maintaining regular contact with your doctor you can keep track of your symptoms and learn to control your thyroid problem.

WHEN SHOULD I SEEK MEDICAL HELP?

Thyroid disorders can often go unnoticed in the early stages, because the symptoms (like weight gain or weight loss) can come on gradually and can be quite subtle at first. It's not just you that may not notice something is out of the ordinary – your close family and friends may see too much of you to notice anything unusual. People who

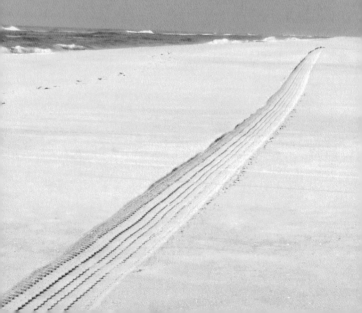

have not seen you for a while (like your doctor) may be more likely to notice these subtle changes. It is probably more likely that your doctor will have detected your thyroid disorder during a routine check-up or when you went to see them about a seemingly unrelated complaint. It may be that you notice your symptoms worsen suddenly or start to affect your lifestyle more than they used to.

If you suspect that something is wrong, it is important that you seek medical advice. Many people who are diagnosed with a thyroid disorder have put up with their symptoms for a while before they finally pluck up the courage to go and see their doctor. It is always best to get these things checked out as soon as possible. Although you may not like what your doctor is telling you, trust their experience and judgement. Try to work with them.

DIAGNOSING THYROID DISORDERS

When you first visit your doctor, he or she will ask you a number of questions about your symptoms and about your health in general. Questions like:

- when did you first notice these symptoms?

- does anything make them better or worse?

- what other types of medication are you taking?

- is there a history of thyroid disease in your family?

- have you ever had surgery on your thyroid gland?

- were you recently pregnant?

They will also take stock of their overall impression of you as you walk into the consultation room. This is important and can provide many clues as to whether or not you have a problem with your thyroid. It may be that they notice tell-tale eye symptoms or perhaps a prominent lump in your throat.

If you do have a visible lump or swelling in your throat (a goitre), your doctor will want to take a closer look at it. They will feel (or palpate) the lump to check whether:

- it is a single lump or multiple lumps

- it has nodules on it

- it is soft or firm

- it is in the region of the thyroid gland

- it moves with swallowing.

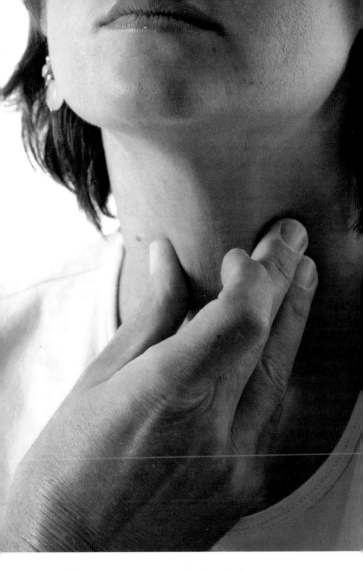

Different types of lump can indicate different types of thyroid disorder. Most lumps are benign (that is to say, not cancerous) but sometimes your doctor may want to make sure by ordering a needle biopsy (to extract tissue for analysis) and/or an ultrasound scan (see page 73).

TESTING THYROID FUNCTION

If your doctor suspects that your symptoms may relate to a problem with your thyroid, he or she may order some blood tests for confirmation and your blood sample will be sent away to a laboratory to be analysed. Your doctor will only order (thyroid) blood tests if your symptoms seem to suggest that you may have a thyroid disorder. They will not order tests indiscriminately because if you have no symptoms then the result of the tests can sometimes be misleading.

But what are they looking for at the laboratory? Technicians will determine the concentration of:

■ thyroid-stimulating hormone (TSH)

■ free thyroxine (fT4)

■ and/or free triiodothyronine (fT3).

This will provide important clues as to how well your thyroid is working. The amount of TSH is usually determined first. If this is normal, fT3 and fT4 are also likely to be normal and the laboratory will not usually measure these levels. However, if the TSH level is abnormal, fT4 and/or fT3 levels may also be checked to help reach a diagnosis.

'Subclinical' describes the early stage of a disease or condition, before symptoms become noticeable.

WHAT DO THYROID TESTS TELL US?

If your level of TSH is **higher** than normal and your levels of fT4 and/or fT3 are **lower** than normal, it may mean that you have **hypothyroidism.**

If your level of TSH is **lower** than normal and your levels of fT4 and/or fT3 are **higher** than normal, it may mean that you have **hyperthyroidism.**

Subclinical hypothyroidism

If your level of TSH is moderately raised but your level of fT4 is normal, you may be diagnosed with subclinical hypothyroidism.

Subclinical hyperthyroidism

If your level of TSH is low but your level of fT4 is normal, you may be diagnosed with subclinical hyperthyroidism.

Test results can vary according to the laboratory they are performed in so your result will be compared with the normal range in that laboratory.

Guide normal values: TSH 0.3–5.5 mu/L; T3 3.9–6.8 pmol/L; T4 12–22 pmol/L.

In general, the more severe your symptoms, the more abnormal your blood test will be. There are some situations where the results of thyroid tests may be misleading or confusing, but your doctor will be able to interpret them. 'Sick thyroid syndrome' is so called because a short-term illness (especially in elderly people) may suppress TSH in a person who has otherwise normal thyroid function.

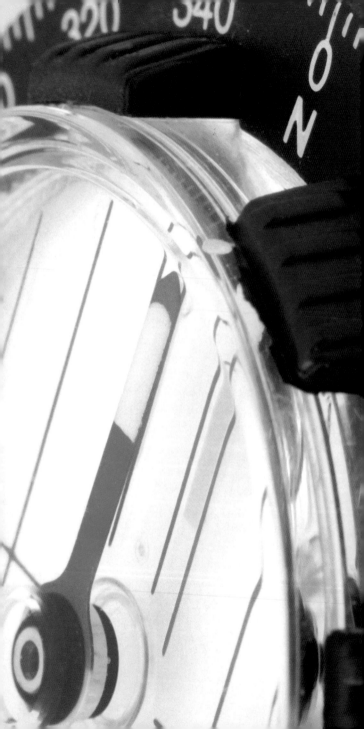

Thyroid medication is not a quick fix...

Some people are very keen to blame their symptoms of tiredness and weight gain on their thyroid gland and actively seek treatment from their doctor. Don't be misled. If your blood tests come back as normal then it is very unlikely that anything is wrong with your thyroid gland.

Your doctor will not recommend thyroid medication if your blood tests come back as normal. It can be dangerous to give the treatment to people who are not suffering from a deficiency of thyroid hormones and can precipitate heart failure, worsen angina, cause atrial fibrillation, worsen diabetes and increase your long-term risk of developing osteoporosis.

How reliable are thyroid tests?

Before jumping to any conclusions, your doctor will probably want to perform another blood test, just to make sure. If you do have something wrong with your thyroid, you may need to remain on medication for the rest of your life, and this is something that is not undertaken lightly. Doctors will usually perform more than one blood test to ensure that the initial diagnosis is correct.

If the blood test results do not fit with what your doctor is expecting to see (going by your symptoms) they may ask you further questions. Drugs like amiodarone ([Cordarone X®, Amyben®] taken for cardiac arrhythmias) and lithium ([Camcolit 400®, Lithonate®, Liskonum®, Priadel®] taken for some psychiatric conditions like bipolar disorder) can sometimes affect the thyroid.

Monitoring your thyroid function

Once you have started treatment, it is important that your thyroid function is retested regularly so that your doctor can judge whether your treatment is working or not. They will probably wait until you have settled into your treatment programme before they order more blood tests. It can take some time for levels of TSH to return to normal and so taking a blood test too early can give misleading results. To start with, you will usually have your thyroid function retested after 5–8 weeks. After this, you will not usually need to be monitored this often.

WILL I BE REFERRED?

Whether or not you are referred to a specialist (called an endocrinologist) largely depends on the results of your initial blood test.

- If the test reveals that you are suffering from **hypothyroidism** then you will only be referred under special circumstances (e.g. if you are a child, if you do not respond well to treatment or if you are pregnant or have just had a baby) and you will usually be managed by your GP.

- If the test reveals that you are suffering from **hyperthyroidism** then you are usually referred to a specialist as a matter of course.

OTHER TESTS

■ **A blood test for thyroid-stimulating autoantibodies**

The presence of elevated levels of these antibodies may (but does not always) indicate autoimmune thyroid disease (like Hashimoto's thyroiditis and Graves' disease). Antibodies can sometimes help to predict whether you will go on to develop thyroid disease.

■ **A blood test to measure cholesterol**

It is recommended that all middle-aged people have their cholesterol levels monitored as a matter of course. Some types of thyroid disorder can affect your cholesterol levels.

■ **A fine needle aspiration (FNA)**

A thin, hollow needle is used to withdraw a sample from a thyroid lump and the contents are examined under a microscope. This can help to identify cancerous cells but is not always 100% reliable.

■ **Ultrasound**

After carefully examining your neck and feeling your thyroid, your specialist may order an ultrasound scan to determine whether goitre is compressing the windpipe or to determine the nature of a nodule.

■ **A CT (computed tomography) scan**

This can be used to work out exactly how far below your collar bone your goitre has gone, and to see if it is pressing on your windpipe. CT scans are often ordered before surgery is considered.

DIAGNOSING THYROID CANCER

If your doctor suspects that you may have thyroid cancer then you will be referred to a specialist straight away. Your doctor may be particularly cautious if there is a history of thyroid cancer running in your family.

Remember that thyroid cancer is extremely rare in the UK and represents only about 1% of all cancers. If you are diagnosed with thyroid cancer there is a very good chance you'll make a full recovery given the right treatment.

Symptoms and signs of thyroid cancer can vary. They may (but do not always) include:

– a lump in the neck that gradually increases in size, with or without pain
– difficulties swallowing or breathing.

The thyroid specialist will carry out many of the thyroid function tests mentioned in the previous pages. If these come back normal then there is more chance that this is not simply a matter of hypo- or hyperthyroidism, although it still doesn't necessarily mean that you have cancer.

The treatment of thyroid cancer is discussed later on in this section (page 112).

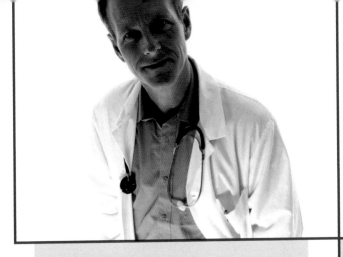

ENDOCRINOLOGIST

I am a hospital doctor specially trained to manage thyroid disorders like hyperthyroidism and thyroid cancer. I will also manage people with hypothyroidism under certain circumstances. You will usually be referred to me by your GP, after a blood test has confirmed that you have a thyroid disorder.

I will tailor your programme of care to suit your individual needs. For hyperthyroidism, treatment may involve antithyroid medication, radioiodine therapy, surgery or a combination of all of these methods. In order to ensure that the course of treatment I recommend is working as it should, I will request regular blood tests and regular check-up appointments. I will communicate directly with your GP, and we will work together to control your thyroid condition.

Radioiodine therapy is usually administered by a specialist called a nuclear medicine technician. The procedure will take place in a specially designated area of the hospital and that the specialist or radiologist looking after you will carefully record exactly how much radiation you receive.

75

THYROID SCREENING

Screening programmes are designed to detect thyroid disorders in susceptible people before they would otherwise have been brought to their (or their doctor's) attention. In an ideal world, everyone would be routinely screened for all manner of diseases. However, this would be extremely expensive and time-consuming (and would be unnecessary in most people). Experts have recommended that the following people should be screened for thyroid disorders as a matter of course:

- people with a strong family history of thyroid disease

- people who have been treated with lithium or amiodarone for prolonged periods

- newborn babies.

In the UK, all newborn babies are routinely screened for hypothyroidism when they are a few days old so that any abnormalities are picked up early and treated accordingly. Your doctor or midwife will take a blood sample by pricking your baby's heel (also called the Guthrie test).

WHAT WILL MY DOCTOR RECOMMEND?

The course of treatment you will be given largely depends on what type of thyroid disorder you have been diagnosed with.

- **Goitre.** Depending on the nature of the swelling, you may be offered surgery or medication or you may not need any treatment at all.

- **Hypothyroidism.** You will usually be offered thyroid hormone replacement therapy.

- **Hyperthyroidism.** You will usually be offered treatment with antithyroid drugs, radioiodine treatment or surgery, or a combination of these.

- **Thyroid cancer.** You will usually have your thyroid removed with surgery followed by a course of radioiodine treatment and thyroid hormone replacement therapy.

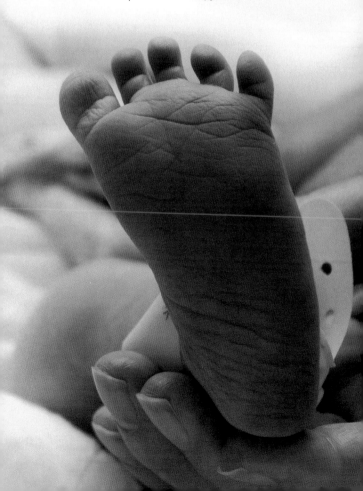

CONCORDANCE

Concordance is the extent to which a person follows the recommendations of their doctor, particularly with respect to taking their medication. Surprisingly, poor concordance is a major issue when it comes to thyroid disorders. But why is this? Nobody knows for sure but it may be because:

- people become complacent if their symptoms are mild enough not to bother them

- people may not want to take medication indefinitely

- people may get confused if they are taking lots of different drugs

- people may simply forget to take their medication.

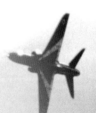

Poor concordance is the most common reason why people have persistently high levels of TSH in their bloodstream despite taking thyroid hormone replacement therapy – they are simply not adhering to the advice their doctor is giving them and not taking their medication as directed.

If you are undergoing thyroid hormone replacement therapy you may be entitled to receive your prescriptions free of charge. Speak to your doctor for more information about this scheme.

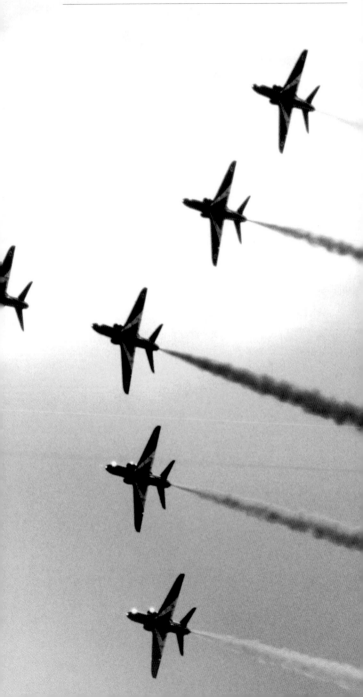

How can I improve my concordance?

■ Undergo regular blood tests (usually annually once you have been stabilised).

■ Listen to your doctor and take on board what he or she is telling you.

■ Be honest. If you forget to take your medication then tell your doctor. This may help to explain some of the symptoms you have been experiencing.

■ Learn about what might happen if you fail to take your medication. Gather and read as much information about thyroid disorders as you can. Of course, reading this book is a great start!

■ Take an active role in the management programme your doctor devises for you and ask lots of questions during your consultations – this is YOUR time.

■ Attend regular check-ups – this gives you a chance to talk about your symptoms and gives your doctor a chance to assess how you are getting on with your treatment.

■ Communicate with other people with thyroid problems and share your experiences with them. Being aware that you're not the only one with a problem can be immensely reassuring (see *Simple extras* page 129).

Arrange your medication next to your toothbrush or teapot so that you remember to take it. You can also ask your GP or pharmacist to reorder your medication at regular intervals.

GIVING UP SMOKING

Whilst smoking may be something that you resort to in times of stress, it is important to try to give up. Aside from the detrimental effects smoking has on your general health, there is a strong link between smoking and the eye problems that are associated with Graves' disease.

People who smoke have the greatest chance of developing severe thyroid eye disease compared with non-smokers. If you are trying to give up, then your local NHS Stop Smoking Service can help by putting you in touch with specially trained advisors (call 0800 169 0169).

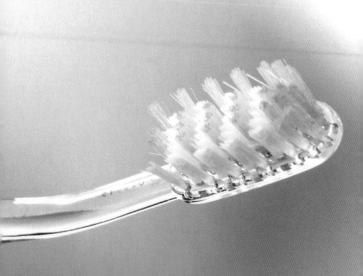

MANAGING YOUR WEIGHT

If you have been diagnosed with a thyroid disorder, it is very likely that you will have experienced some degree of fluctuation in your weight. This may even be the reason why you first sought medical advice. Eating a healthy balanced diet and exercising regularly can help you to control your weight. Once your thyroid disorder has been treated, your weight will tend to go back to where it was before.

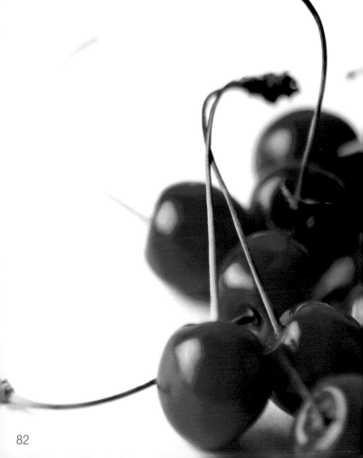

Following a healthy, balanced diet means eating:

- more fruit, vegetables and salad
- two portions of fish per week
- less saturated fat substitute with mono- and poly-unsaturated fats, including omega-3 fats (found in fish oils and oily fish like mackerel and sardines)
- fresh rather than processed foods
- less salt (no more than 6 g salt per day [about a teaspoon])
- less sugary foods (less refined sugar [the white sugar used to sweeten and preserve food])
- more fibre (found in wholegrain starchy foods and beans, peas, lentils).

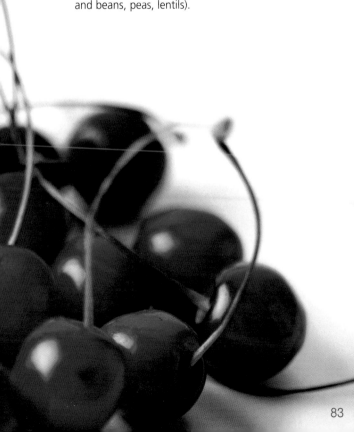

MANAGING GOITRE

There are many types of goitre (e.g. solitary nodule, multinodular, smooth, unilateral [affecting only one side of the thyroid] or bilateral [affecting both sides]) and the most appropriate course of treatment depends on the exact nature of the goitre you are diagnosed with. If your goitre is not malignant, is relatively small or it is not causing you any symptoms, then your specialist may feel that it is best left as it is. If your goitre is large and unsightly then your doctor may recommend that you undergo surgery to have it removed. Before embarking on any treatment approach, your doctor will first check the levels of thyroid hormones in your bloodstream to see if you have underlying hypo- or hyperthyroidism. If this is found to be the case then they may prescribe thyroid hormone replacement therapy or antithyroid drugs (depending on the nature of your thyroid disorder) to help correct the balance of these hormones.

Triple assessment

When dealing with goitre, it is important to determine whether any lump is benign or malignant. Doctors often use the triple assessment procedure to help do this. Triple assessment involves:

- examination
- fine needle aspiration to detect cancerous cells, or to empty cysts of their fluid
- ultrasound.

Three strikes and it's out

Sometimes, completely aspirating the fluid from a
thyroid cyst until all of its contents have been
removed and it can be considered 'dry', is enough
to get rid of it permanently. However, cysts like
this can reappear with time and will need further
aspiration. If the cyst recurs after three such
aspirations then your doctor will probably
recommend that you undergo surgery to have it
removed. This is known as the 'three strikes and
it's out' approach.

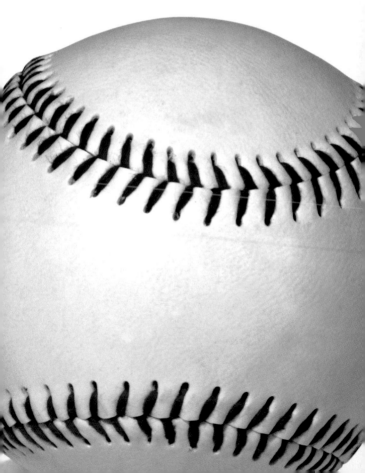

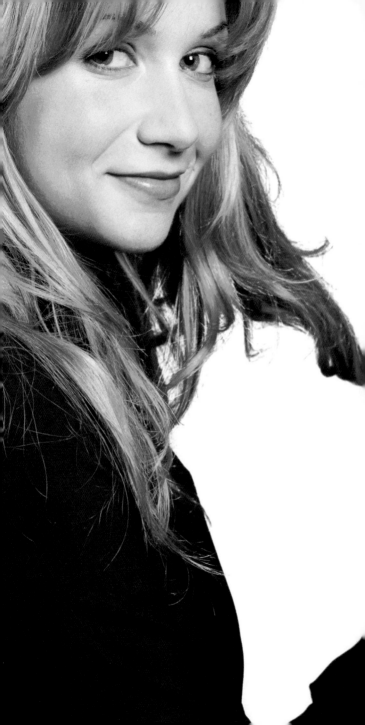

MANAGING HYPOTHYROIDISM

If your thyroid gland is underactive then your doctor will probably recommend that you start taking synthetic **thyroid hormones** to boost the levels of thyroid hormones in your bloodstream, restore the natural balance and get things back to normal. The term synthetic means that these hormones are made in the laboratory (from natural products).

You may also be prescribed this 'thyroid hormone replacement therapy' if you have undergone surgery on your thyroid (or if it has become underactive following radioiodine therapy) in order to control your body's metabolism and do the job that your thyroid gland would otherwise have done.

Your doctor will usually be able to manage your hypothyroidism in your local surgery and you will not normally have to see a specialist. Once you have been diagnosed and prescribed hormone therapy, you will usually have to keep taking it for the rest of your life. Try to make taking your medication part of your daily routine. This way, you won't forget to take it.

Your thyroid function will gradually return to normal. This will not happen overnight and some symptoms (like changes in hair and nails) can take a few weeks to disappear. Once your levels are back to normal, your doctor will probably recommend that you have a blood test once a year to check that your TSH levels remain normal.

■ Levothyroxine sodium

This is also known as thyroxine (T4) and is the most frequently used thyroid replacement hormone in the UK. The body converts it to T3 just as it would if the thyroid gland were producing its own thyroxine. It is almost always taken as a tablet once a day. It can take some time to get the dose of thyroxine right, so your doctor will usually start with a low dose and build it up gradually over a period of weeks to the full replacement dose (approximately 125 µg per day).

If you are elderly or suffer from more than one type of illness, then your doctor will usually want to increase the dose of medication more slowly. If your thyroid is only moderately underactive then you will not usually require the full replacement dose and may be controlled at doses of 50, 75 or 100 µg per day.

Under these circumstances, you will need to undergo a blood test after 6 months to make sure that the dose you are taking is sufficient to control your thyroid disorder, and then again at yearly intervals thereafter.

■ Liothyronine sodium (Tertroxin®; T3)

This works in the same way as thyroxine but is generally reserved for the initial treatment of very severe cases of hypothyroidism, usually as an inpatient in a hospital setting, when it is important to increase thyroid hormones quickly. It can also be given as an injection in very extreme cases. This T3 treatment can also be used to help prepare people for radioiodine therapy during treatment for thyroid cancer.

NATURAL THYROID HORMONE

So-called 'natural thyroid hormones' are made from desiccated (dried) animal thyroid glands rather than being produced synthetically, like the thyroid hormones you will be prescribed on the NHS. Although they are widely available in the USA, most doctors and specialists in this country would advise against the use of natural thyroid hormones in the management of hypothyroidism. There is now reasonable purification, and standardisation of the relevant amounts of T3 and T4 in the preparation, but the ratio may not suit everyone. This treatment does need to be taken two or three times daily.

Side-effects associated with thyroid hormones

People usually feel much better once they are taking thyroid hormones. Side-effects are unusual because a missing hormone is simply being replaced. A few people report heart palpitations, muscle cramps, diarrhoea, vomiting, headache, restlessness and excessive sweating whilst they are taking thyroid hormones. If you do experience unusual symptoms it may be because you are taking too much. Consult your doctor if these symptoms persist.

Although thyroid medications have been used for over 50 years and doctors are very experienced at using them, no drug treatment is without side-effects. People may respond in slightly different ways to the same medicine. If you experience symptoms which you think may be due to the thyroid, or indeed any other medication you are taking, you should always talk to your doctor, pharmacist or nurse. If the side-effect is unusual or severe, your GP may decide to report it to the Medicines and Healthcare products Regulatory Agency (MHRA). The MHRA operates a 'Yellow Card Scheme' which is designed to flag up potentially dangerous drug effects and thereby protect your safety. The procedure has changed recently to allow patients to report adverse drug reactions themselves. Visit *www.yellowcard.gov.uk* for more information. You should always ask your doctor if you are concerned about any aspect of your management plan.

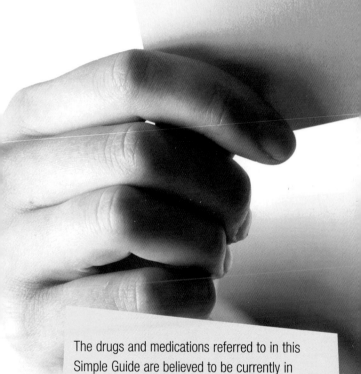

The drugs and medications referred to in this Simple Guide are believed to be currently in widespread use in the UK. Medical science can evolve rapidly, but to the best of our knowledge, this is a reasonable reflection of clinical practice at the time of going to press.

Source: British National Formulary.

MANAGING SUBCLINICAL HYPOTHYROIDISM

As we have seen, subclinical hypothyroidism is borderline hypothyroidism. A blood test may reveal a slight abnormality in the levels of your thyroid hormones but you may not be experiencing any symptoms. In this instance, the dilemma faced by doctors is whether or not to treat you. Many cases of subclinical hypothyroidism resolve by themselves and there is no need for treatment.

Doctors can vary in their approach. Some prefer to offer treatment. Others recommend frequent blood tests to see whether full-blown hypothyroidism (with symptoms) does indeed develop. If your TSH blood test is persistently abnormal then you are more likely to be offered thyroid hormone replacement treatment. As mentioned earlier, the presence of thyroid antibodies in your bloodstream can sometimes indicate that you are likely to develop a thyroid disorder later on, and so this test may be useful in people with subclinical disease.

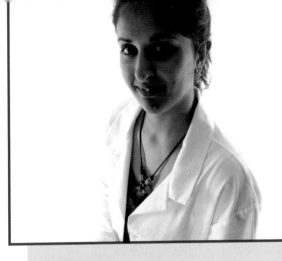

PHARMACIST

As a pharmacist within the Primary Care Trust, I offer people essential services like drug dispensing and self-care support, usually within their local area. I can also provide you with lifestyle advice (such as what to include in a healthy diet and how to manage your weight). Pharmacists within the community now play a bigger role than ever before in helping people to manage their conditions. This may involve keeping track of which medications you are using and how often.

A number of new schemes have been laid out in our new pharmacy contract, which reflects the government's health priorities: support for self-care, management of long-term conditions and public health. By increasing the range of services that we can offer, we can improve the level of care and support that you, as a patient with a long-term condition like a thyroid disorder, can expect from your health service.

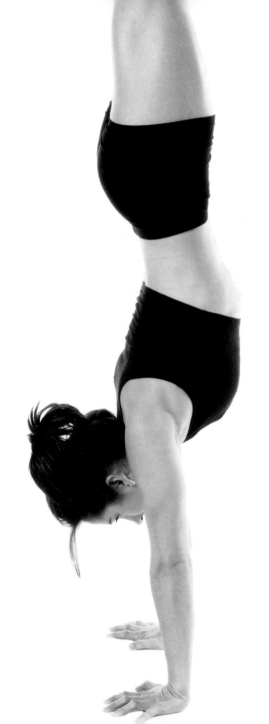

MANAGING HYPERTHYROIDISM

If your thyroid gland is producing too many thyroid hormones then there are a number of different treatment options your doctor or specialist may recommend in order to restore the natural balance and get things back to normal. In a minority of cases, hyperthyroidism sorts itself out, but most people need treatment. The most common management approaches for hyperthyroidism are described below. They include antithyroid drug treatment, radioiodine or surgery. Sometimes your doctor will recommend a combination of one or more strategies.

Antithyroid drugs

Antithyroid drugs work by slowing down the manufacture of thyroid hormones by the thyroid gland. Your doctor or specialist may decide that your hyperthyroidism can be managed with drug treatment. They may also sometimes recommend that you take these medications to prepare you for thyroid surgery. You may also be prescribed antithyroid drugs in conjunction with radioiodine treatment.

With hyperthyroidism, you will not necessarily need to take medication indefinitely (as is the case for hypothyroidism) – treatment with these drugs is usually for 18 months or longer. Shorter periods of treatment are associated with a higher likelihood of symptom relapse.

Dose titration

It is important to get the dose of antithyroid medication correct because if it is too high, it may cause hypothyroidism – the other extreme. The gradual adjustment of dosage is called dose titration. Regular thyroid blood tests (carried out every 6 and then every 8 weeks) are used to check that the dose of antithyroid drug is correct.

Carbimazole (Neo-Mercazole®) and propylthiouracil are the two antithyroid drugs currently available in the UK. Carbimazole tends to be used more often. Treatment at the starting dose (20–40 mg per day) usually continues for 6–8 weeks until thyroid function returns to normal, and then the dosage is gradually reduced to a 'maintenance dose' of between 10 and 15 mg per day (and thyroid blood tests are used to make sure that thyroid function remains under control). Propylthiouracil is usually given at a starting dose of 200–400 mg per day, reducing to a daily maintenance dose of between 100 and 150 mg. If you are pregnant you are more likely to be treated with propylthiouracil. Treatment with these drugs usually continues for 18 months or longer.

The block–replace regimen

Your specialist may recommend the 'block–replace regimen' to control your hyperthyroidism. This involves completely suppressing the natural output of the thyroid gland using high doses of antithyroid drugs and using thyroid hormone replacement therapy (the T4 tablets that are used to treat hypothyroidism) as the only source of thyroid hormones in the body. This approach is not favoured by all endocrinologists, although there is evidence that it works well and may be beneficial in certain situations such as significant thyroid eye disease.

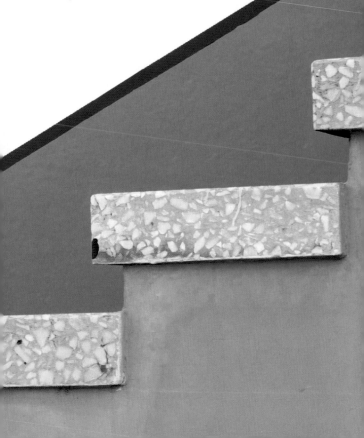

Side-effects associated with antithyroid drugs

Whilst most people who take antithyroid drugs get on very well with them, there are a few side-effects you should watch out for. A fever, mouth ulcers and sore throats can all indicate a condition called agranulocytosis – a potentially dangerous reduction in the number of white blood cells within the body. If you notice any of these symptoms you should contact your doctor or specialist immediately as a matter of course.

A small proportion of people develop an itchy red skin rash shortly after they start taking antithyroid drugs. If the rash persists, you should stop taking the medication and consult your doctor immediately.

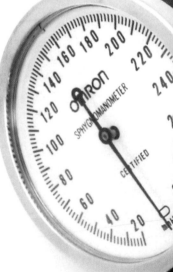

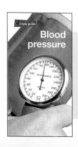

For more information see
Blood pressure

Beta-blockers and hyperthyroidism

Beta-blockers (like propanolol) are drugs that work by controlling the effects of the hormone adrenaline (which include stress, tremor, sweating, palpitations and feeling hot). They are often used to treat high blood pressure (hypertension). People with hyperthyroidism tend to be more sensitive to adrenaline and so often find that taking a beta-blocker can help to control some of their symptoms. You will usually only be given a beta-blocker for a few weeks at most and not normally if you have asthma.

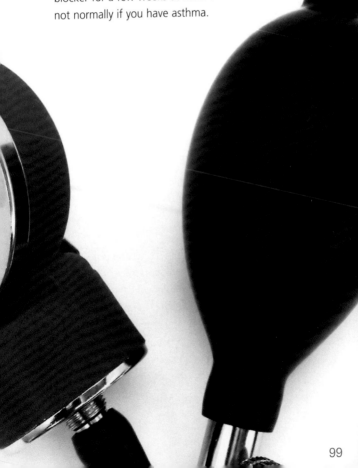

Radioiodine

If you have failed to respond to antithyroid medication, your specialist will probably recommend that you undergo treatment with radioiodine. This is a commonly used treatment approach for hyperthyroidism. If you are pregnant, intending to become pregnant or breast-feeding you will not be given radioiodine (see later in the section, page 114).

Radioiodine is iodine that is radioactive. When the radioiodine is given as a capsule or drink, it is automatically taken up by the thyroid gland as a raw material for the manufacture of T3 or T4. As the radioactivity builds up in the thyroid gland, it destroys some of the thyroid tissue. It is important that the radiologist (or specialist or specially-trained doctor) uses exactly the right amount of radiation (enough to return thyroid function to normal but not so much that the thyroid gland is destroyed completely). Striking exactly the right balance (or hitting the bullseye!) is difficult and some people will end up needing to take thyroid hormone replacement therapy to combat hypothyroidism after the procedure.

Generally speaking, the higher the dose of radioiodine you receive, the greater your chance of developing hypothyroidism over the weeks/months/years following the procedure. If you have had radioiodine therapy in the past, you will have yearly thyroid function tests even if your thyroid is apparently functioning normally without hormone replacement therapy.

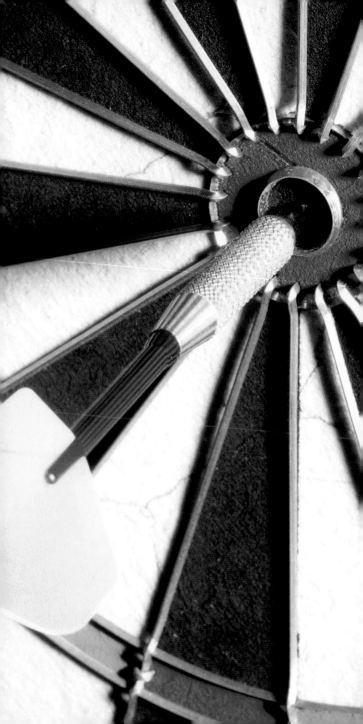

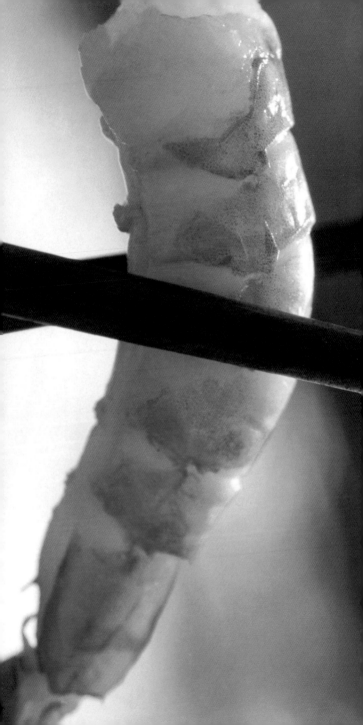

You will be told to stop taking your thyroid hormones for about 2 weeks before the procedure because these will interfere with how well the radioiodine is taken up by the thyroid gland. You may also be told to avoid foods that contain high levels of iodine (like seafood, seaweed and some vegetables).

Is it dangerous?

Radioiodine is not dangerous when it is given in small quantities in the controlled manner described previously. However, it is very important that you (or the healthcare professional treating you) are not exposed to any more radiation than is absolutely necessary. This is why the procedure will take place in a specially designated area of the hospital and that the radiologist looking after you will carefully record exactly how much radiation you receive. You may also be told to avoid close contact with pregnant women or young children for a couple of weeks after the procedure so that you do not inadvertently expose them to radiation (your specialist will discuss this with you). If you have had radioiodine treatment for thyroid cancer, you may have to stay in hospital until the radiologist is satisfied that the bulk of the radioactivity has left your body in your urine.

MANAGING GRAVES' DISEASE

Since Graves' disease is a type of hyperthyroidism, it will usually be managed in much the same way to that described previously. The most common approach is to use the antithyroid drug, carbimazole. However, as we have seen, Graves' disease is often associated with a number of symptoms that affect the eyes. This occurs when the autoimmune response affects not only the thyroid gland but spills over to the cells behind the eyeball and makes them swell up, forcing the eyeball outwards. Currently, it is unclear why some people with Graves' disease develop thyroid eye disease and others do not.

For some people with Graves' disease, radioiodine treatment is not appropriate because it can worsen their eye problems (especially in people who smoke). It is difficult to predict who will react badly to it though so most specialists choose to proceed with caution.

If you do suffer from Graves' ophthalmopathy it is advisable that you attend regular check-ups with a specialised ophthalmologist to keep track of the changes occurring with your vision.

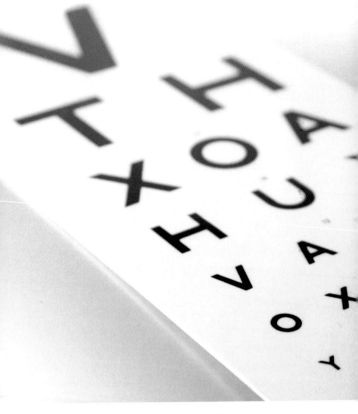

You may find that the following help on a
day-to-day basis.

- Giving up smoking.
- Wrap-around sunglasses to help protect light-
  sensitive eyes from glare and limit wind-drying
  of the eyes.
- Special prism glasses that help to correct
  double vision.
- Eye drops and ointments to lubricate dry eyes.
- Humidifiers to keep the atmosphere around
  you moist and less irritating to your eyes.
- Elevating your head whilst you are asleep.

If you suffer from very severe Graves' ophthalmopathy you may be given high doses of steroid drugs, which act as anti-inflammatory agents and keep the swelling around the eyes under control. However, this is not a long-term solution because very high doses of these drugs can cause weight gain and thinning of the bones and skin. In order to counteract the effects of these steroids, you may also be given antiosteoporosis medication (e.g. alendronic acid, disodium etidronate, disodium pamidronate, strontium ranelate, ibandronic acid) to protect your bones and a proton pump inhibitor (e.g. lansoprazole, omeprazole) to reduce the risk of peptic ulcers. At times the immunosuppressant azathioprine (Azamune®, Immunoprin®) can also be given to help limit the amount of steroid you need to take.

A fairly major operation called orbital decompression is used to remove some of the bone surrounding the eye in order to give the swollen eye muscles more room to move and bring down the swelling. Another technique, now more commonly performed than surgery is called orbital radiotherapy and can be used to reduce the amount of inflammation affecting the fatty tissue behind the eye and also the small muscles that move the eyeball.

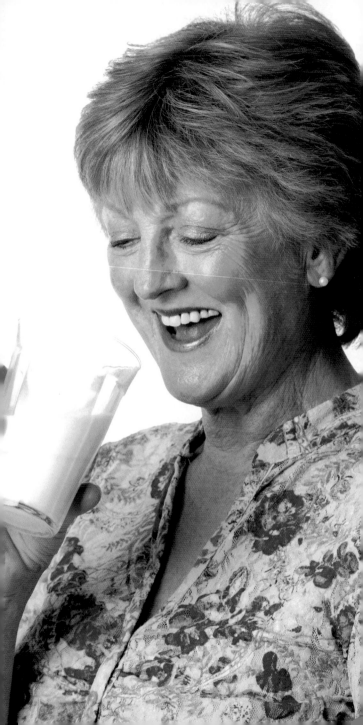

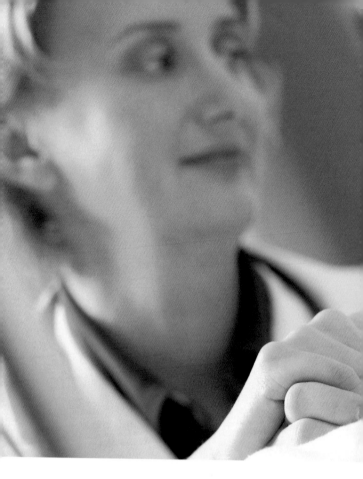

MANAGING THYROID DISORDERS WITH SURGERY

Sometimes, your specialist will opt surgically to remove your thyroid gland. Sometimes, if the goitre is one-sided, your surgeon will opt to remove only one of the thyroid lobes with a thyroid lobectomy (usually taking the isthmus too [an isthmectomy]). The tissue from the removed lobe is quickly examined under a microscope to see if there may be a malignant risk and if there is, the rest of the thyroid is taken out during the same operation. This is called a thyroidectomy. You are more likely to be referred for surgery if:

- you are young
- you have a large goitre that is starting to restrict your swallowing or breathing
- drug treatment has failed to improve your hyperthyroidism or you are allergic to the thyroid medication
- your specialist suspects that you may have thyroid cancer (see page 112).

So what happens after the surgery?

- If you have had your thyroid gland removed completely then you will have to take thyroid hormone replacement therapy for the rest of your life. Your doctor will regularly monitor your thyroid function by performing blood tests.
- If only part of the thyroid is removed then you may not need hormone replacement therapy – a blood test will confirm whether you need this or not.
- You'll probably have to stay in hospital for about 3 days afterwards and you may need to take a few weeks off work, depending on your occupation.
- Your surgeon (and your specialist) will probably want to see you at least once during the weeks after your operation.

'Ectomy' is a suffix added to the end of a word that means 'surgical removal' of the affected part.

What are the risks associated with thyroid surgery?

Thyroid surgery is carried out under a general anaesthetic and usually takes around 2 hoursto complete. The success rate of surgery is very high and most people can expect to return to normal thyroid functioning afterwards. Of course, no operation is without its risks, and very rarely, damage to the nerves supplying the vocal cords can occur. This usually only causes temporary hoarseness. If, as rarely can occur, your parathyroid glands are damaged during the operation, you may have to take long-term calcium and vitamin D supplements. Tingling sensations in your hands, fingers, toes and lips in the days after your operation can mean that you have low levels of calcium in your blood. The surgeon will arrange for your vocal cords and calcium levels to be checked both before and after surgery.

It is important that you understand what your specialist is proposing to do – make sure that you ask plenty of questions like:

- what are the risks associated with this procedure?
- what is the success rate?
- how long will I have to remain in hospital?
- how much time will I need to take off work?
- will I still have to take medication even after the operation?
- how long have you been doing this procedure and how many do you do in a year?

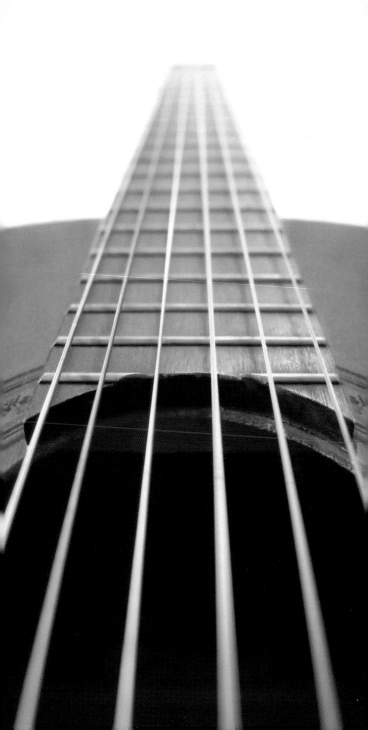

THE TREATMENT OF THYROID CANCER

If the tests performed on your suspect thyroid lump confirm that you have thyroid cancer then your specialist will work quickly to arrange a programme of treatment. With the modern treatments now available, the outlook for people with cancer of the thyroid is very good and most people are completely cured.

You should be kept well informed of what's happening and you may be offered counselling by a trained nurse specialist. Your GP will also be kept informed of all your test results so you should feel free to go and discuss any concerns you may have with him or her. Your specialist will probably recommend the following course of treatment.

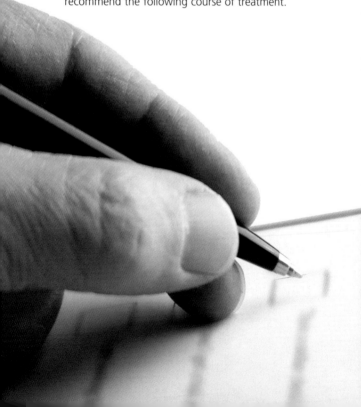

1. A total thyroidectomy (see page 108) to remove your thyroid gland (taking the cancerous tissue with it).
2. Radioiodine treatment to destroy any remaining cancer cells (may also be used to treat thyroid cancer that has spread to other parts of the body).
3. Thyroid hormone replacement therapy for the rest of your life.
4. Regular scans and blood tests to check that the cancer has not returned.

Block neck dissection

Sometimes, a malignant thyroid mass can also affect the lymph nodes. These are the bean-shaped structures of the immune system that remove cell waste and help the body to fight infections. If the lymph nodes are involved, these and adjacent tissues will be removed at the same time, in what is termed a block neck dissection. Under these circumstances, an ear nose and throat surgeon will often join the endocrine surgeon for the operation.

MANAGING A THYROID DISORDER DURING PREGNANCY AND AFTER GIVING BIRTH

If you are pregnant or breast-feeding then your thyroid disorder will probably be handled slightly differently.

Hypothyroidism

If you have hypothyroidism, it is important that it is managed properly whilst you are pregnant. Poorly controlled hypothyroidism can be associated with maternal anaemia (a low red blood cell count), pre-eclampsia (high blood pressure that causes severe swelling and carries risk for both the mother and the unborn baby) and a low birth weight.

■ If you need it, you will be prescribed thyroid hormone replacement therapy as normal (although some women may require a higher dose than usual). Taking these hormone tablets will not put your unborn baby at risk.

■ Your doctor will monitor your thyroid function with regular blood tests.

■ You will still be able to breast-feed whilst taking thyroid hormones.

Hyperthyroidism

Again, if it is not managed properly, hyperthyroidism carries significant risks for both you and your baby, sometimes leading to early labour and pre-eclampsia.

■ If your hyperthyroidism is mild, you will probably be monitored closely without treatment.

■ There is no evidence to suggest that the antithyroid medications, carbimazole and propylthiouracil, are harmful to pregnant women or their unborn children. You will not be offered the block–replace regimen whilst you are pregnant.

■ If you have severe hyperthyroidism then your doctor will normally advise you against trying to get pregnant until it is under control.

■ You will not be given radioiodine therapy. This is because the thyroid gland of the growing foetus would absorb the radioactive iodine and could become damaged as a result.

■ You may be offered surgery if you do not respond to drug treatment but this is not usually recommended owing to the risks to the mother and foetus associated with general anaesthesia. If surgery is appropriate it will usually be carried out in the middle trimester of your pregnancy.

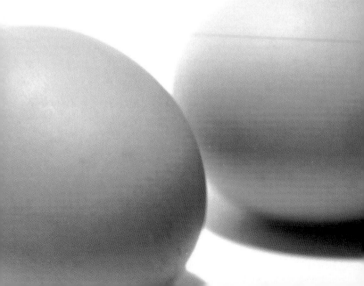

Graves' disease and pregnancy

This is the most common cause of hyperthyroidism experienced during pregnancy. If you have Graves' disease, the chances are that it will worsen in the first 3 months after giving birth. You may need to take higher doses of antithyroid medication during this period and your doctor will want to monitor your thyroid function closely. Breast-feeding is possible if you are receiving moderate (e.g. up to 20 mg of carbimazole) doses of antithyroid drugs but close monitoring of thyroid function, both in the mother and the child, is necessary.

Transient thyrotoxicosis post-partum

This is a form of temporary hyperthyroidism that can affect some women after they have given birth. It occurs up to 12 weeks after delivery. The symptoms of transient thyrotoxicosis are usually relatively mild and are managed by a short course of beta-blockers. You may experience a recurrence during future pregnancies.

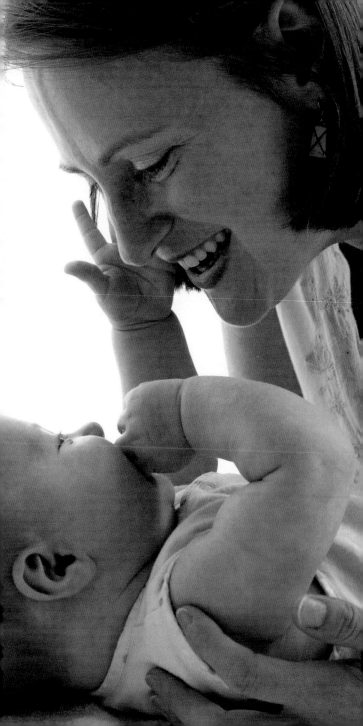

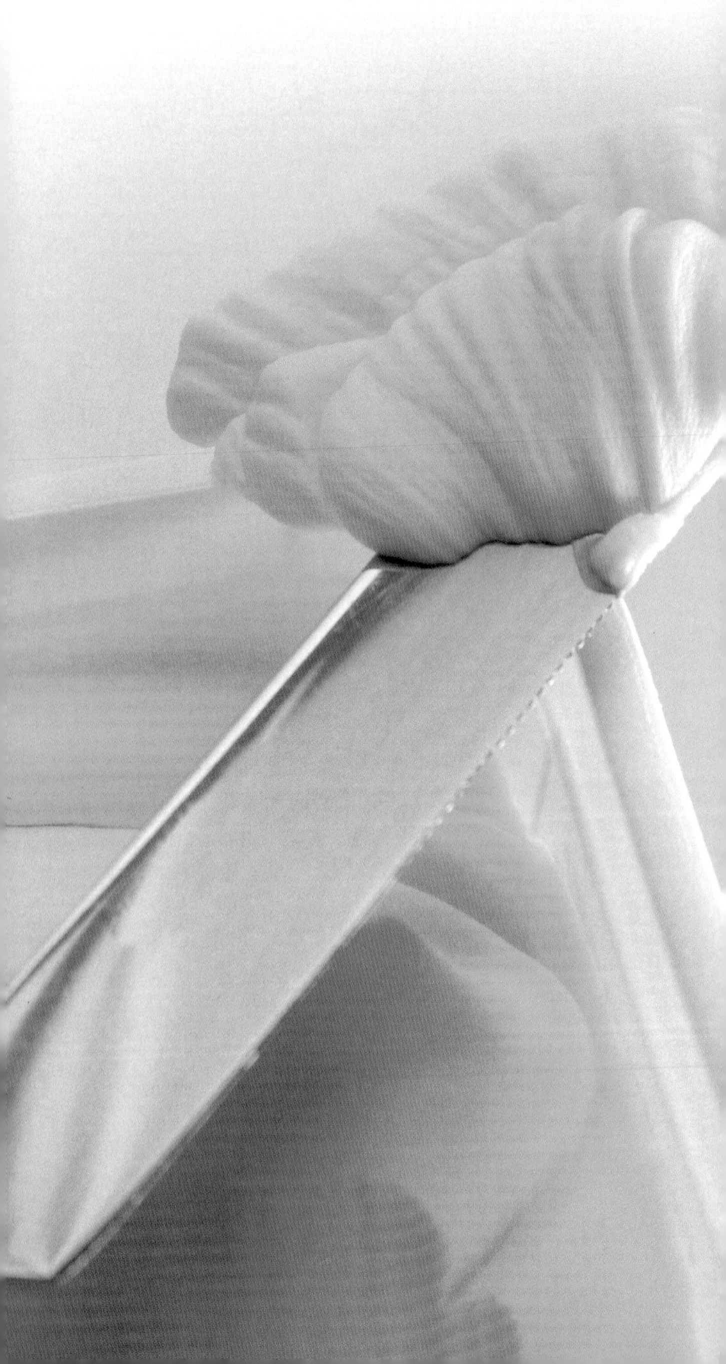

THYROID DISORDERS AND HEART DISEASE

As we have seen, thyroid disorders can sometimes affect the heart, causing palpitations, chest pain, or even heart failure. These symptoms are much more likely to occur in people with thyroid disorders who have underlying heart disease from another cause. In some people, low thyroxine levels can lead to an increase in blood cholesterol levels which if left unchecked for many years, can increase their risk of developing coronary heart disease.

It is therefore important that the level of thyroxine in the blood is corrected in people who are particularly at risk from heart disease. For these people it is important that treatment with thyroid hormones is initiated gradually.

MANAGING A THYROID DISORDER IN THE ELDERLY

Thyroid disorders tend to be more common in the elderly, although they can sometimes be mistaken for other illnesses and the symptoms can be slightly unusual which can complicate the diagnosis. The treatment of hypothyroidism in the elderly is no different from the standard as far as choice of drug is concerned. However, thyroid replacement is usually introduced more gradually in severely hypothyroid elderly than in younger people. For hyperthyroidism, radioiodine is usually the treatment of choice in elderly people.

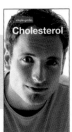

For more information see
Cholesterol

COMPLEMENTARY TREATMENTS

Some non-conventional treatments may help to improve your thyroid symptoms, although there is of course no guarantee that they will work. These treatments should always be used in concert with conventional medicine and should never substitute for the programme of care your doctor or specialist is recommending.

Always proceed with caution when dealing with herbal supplements and use them in strict accordance with their instructions. Claims regarding their effectiveness and safety are generally not reinforced by well-designed clinical trials performed in lots of people (this is in contrast to drugs, which have to go through strict testing procedures before they can be widely used in people).

Inform your doctor if you are considering a complementary treatment. They will be able to advise you what's appropriate and may even be able to put you in touch with a qualified practitioner.

Kelp, a type of iodine-rich seaweed, is not generally recommended by doctors. Ingesting too much iodine (without medical supervision) can sometimes bring on a more severe form of hyperthyroidism and rarely, this can lead to thyroid crisis (a rapid worsening of hyperthyroidism that may lead to life-threatening heart problems).

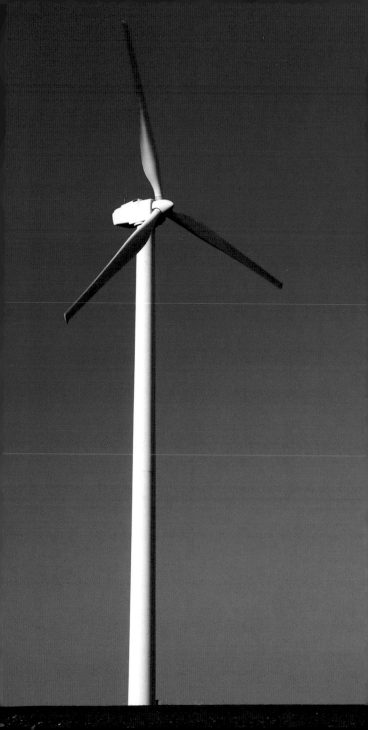

THE LONG AND THE SHORT OF IT

Thyroid disorders affect different people in different ways. The symptoms you experience will probably differ considerably from those of a friend or relative diagnosed with a similar problem. If your thyroid disorder is properly managed it should not end up dictating what you can and can't do and it will not shorten your life expectancy.

Getting your thyroid disorder diagnosed is the first positive step you can take. Thyroid disorders, no matter how mild or severe, can be managed extremely well with the medications and other treatments that we have available these days. Whether you are managed by your GP at your local surgery or referred to a thyroid specialist, be assured that you are in the best possible hands. Listen to what they tell you, take it seriously and try to adhere to the programme of care that they are recommending. It is YOUR responsibility to remember to take your medication every day and to attend your scheduled check-ups, not your doctor's. This is very important, even if your symptoms stop bothering you after a while.

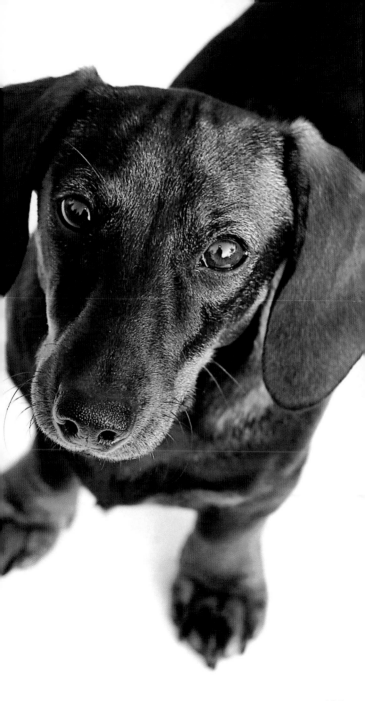

GETTING THE MOST OUT OF YOUR HEALTH SERVICE

As we saw earlier – concordance is a major issue in thyroid disorders. It is vitally important that you take your medication as directed by your doctor, even during those times when your symptoms are not bothering you particularly. If you forget to take your medication, be honest with your doctor and tell them. This will help him or her to work out why your treatment may not be working as they would have hoped.

How you can help your health service to help you

- Don't be afraid to keep going back to your doctor if you don't see any positive changes in your symptoms. Remember though that it can take quite some time for your symptoms to improve.
- Stay in regular contact. Report any worsening of symptoms or side-effects of treatment to your doctor immediately.
- Take all your pills or list to the specialist consultation.
- Ask your doctor to explain any advice they give you. Understanding why something should improve your symptoms can really help you get to grips with your thyroid disorder. Many specialists will be happy to let you have a copy of the letter they send to your GP.
- See if a self-help support group exists in your local area and get involved (see *Simple extras* page 129).

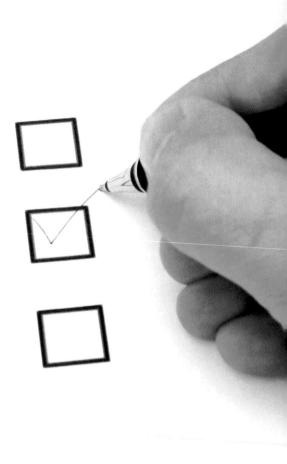

Visiting your doctor or any healthcare professional can sometimes be a confusing or daunting prospect. You may find that the consultation flies by and when your doctor asks if you have any questions, your mind goes blank. Writing down a list of questions before the consultation may help you to get the most out of your appointment.

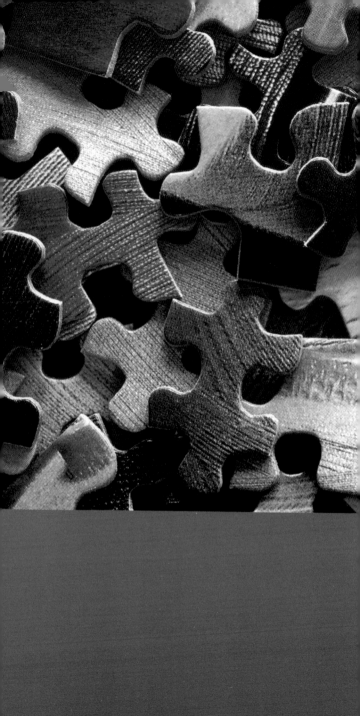

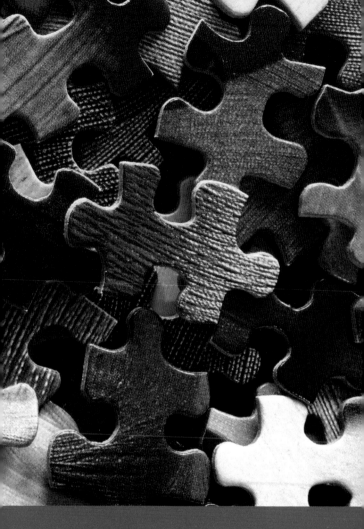

Simple
extras

FURTHER READING

■ *Blood pressure (Simple Guide)*
CSF Medical Communications Ltd, 2005
ISBN: 1-905466-04-8, £5.99
www.bestmedicine.com

■ *Cholesterol (Simple Guide)*
CSF Medical Communications Ltd, 2005
ISBN: 1-905466-05-6, £5.99
www.bestmedicine.com

■ *Arthritis (Simple Guide)*
CSF Medical Communications Ltd, 2006
ISBN: 1-905466-12-9, £5.99
www.bestmedicine.com

■ *Menopause (Simple Guide)*
CSF Medical Communications Ltd, 2006
ISBN: 1-905466-13-7, £5.99
www.bestmedicine.com

USEFUL CONTACTS

■ **British Association of Endocrine Surgeons**
Royal College of Surgeons
35-43 Lincoln's Inn Fields
London
WC2A 3PE
Tel: 0207 304 4771
Website: *www.baes.info*

■ **British Association for Counselling and Psychotherapy**
BACP House
35–37 Albert Street
Rugby
Warwickshire
CV21 2SG
Tel: 0870 443 5252
Website: *www.bacp.co.uk*

■ **British Nutrition Foundation**
High Holborn House
52–54 High Holborn
London
WC1V 6RQ
Tel: 020 7404 6504
Email: *postbox@nutrition.org.uk*
Website: *www.nutrition.org.uk*

■ **British Thyroid Association**
Website: *www.british-thyroid-association.org*

■ **British Thyroid Foundation**
PO Box 97
Clifford
Wetherby
West Yorkshire
LS23 6XD
Tel: 01423 709707
Website: *www.btf-thyroid.org*

■ **Cancer Research UK**
PO Box 123
Lincoln's Inn Fields
London
WC2A 3PX
Tel: 020 7121 6699
Website: *www.cancerresearchuk.org*

■ **NHS Smoking Adviceline:** 0800 1690169

■ **Thyroid Eye Disease Charitable Trust**
PO Box 2954
Calne
SN11 8WR
Tel: 0844 8008133
Email: *ted@tedct.co.uk*
Website: *www.tedct.co.uk*

YOUR RIGHTS

As a patient, you have a number of important rights. These include the right to the best possible standard of care, the right to information, the right to dignity and respect, the right to confidentiality and underpinning all of these, the right to good health.

Occasionally, you may feel as though your rights have been compromised, or you may be unsure of where you stand when it comes to qualifying for certain treatments or services. In these instances, there are a number of organisations you can turn to for help and advice. Remember that lodging a complaint against your health service should not compromise the quality of care you receive, either now or in the future.

■ **The Patients Association**
The Patients Association (*www.patients-association.com*) is a UK charity which represents patient rights, influences health policy and campaigns for better patient care.
Contact details:
PO Box 935
Harrow
Middlesex
HA1 3YJ
Helpline: 0845 6084455
Email: *mailbox@patients-association.com*

■ **Citizens Advice Bureau**
The Citizens Advice Bureau (*www.nacab.org.uk*) provides free, independent and confidential advice to NHS patients at a number of outreach centres located throughout the country (*www.adviceguide.org.uk*).
Contact details:
Find your local Citizens Advice Bureau using the search tool at *www.citizensadvice.org.uk.*

■ **Patient Advice and Liaison Services (PALS)**

Set up by the Department of Health (*www.dh.gov.uk*), PALS provide information, support and confidential advice to patients, families and their carers.

Contact details:

Phone your local hospital, clinic, GP surgery or health centre and ask for details of the PALS, or call NHS Direct on 0845 46 47.

■ **The Independent Complaints Advocacy Service (ICAS)**

ICAS is an independent service that can help you bring about formal complaints against your NHS practitioner. ICAS provides support, help, advice and advocacy from experienced advisors and caseworkers.

Contact details:

ICAS Central Team

Myddelton House

115–123 Pentonville Road

London N1 9LZ

Email: *icascentralteam@citizensadvice.org.uk*

Or contact your local ICAS office direct.

Accessing your medical records

You have a legal right to see all your health records under the Data Protection Act of 1998. You can usually make an informal request to your doctor and you should be given access within 40 days. Note that you may have to pay a small fee for the privilege.

You can be denied access to your records if your doctor believes that the information contained within them could cause serious harm to you or another person. If you are applying for access on behalf of someone else, then you will not be granted access to information which the patient gave to his or her doctor on the understanding that it would remain confidential.

Regional Public Services Ombudsmen

■ **The Health Service Ombudsman for England**
Millbank Tower
Millbank
London
SW1P 4QP
Tel: 0845 015 4033 (Minicom 020 7217 4066)
Email: *phso.enquiries@ombudsman.org.uk*
Website: *www.ombudsman.org.uk*

■ **The Public Services Ombudsman for Wales**
1 Ffordd yr Hen Gae
Pencoed
CF35 5LJ
Tel: 01656 641 150
Email: *ask@ombudsman-wales.org.uk*
Website: *www.ombudsman-wales.org*

■ **The Scottish Public Services Ombudsman**
4 Melville Street
Edinburgh
EH3 7NS
Tel: 0870 011 5378 (Text: 0790 049 4372)
Email: *enquiries@scottishombudsman.org.uk*
Website: *www.scottishombudsman.org.uk*

■ **Northern Ireland Ombudsman**
Freepost
BEL 1478
Belfast BT1 6BR
Tel: 0800 343424 (free) or 028 9023 3821
Email: *ombudsman@ni-ombudsman.org.uk*
Website: *www.ni-ombudsman.org.uk*

PERSONAL RECORD:

My Simple Guide

This Simple Guide belongs to:

Name:

Address:

Tel:

Email:

In case of emergency please contact:

Name:

Address:

Tel:

Email:

My Healthcare Team

GP surgery address and telephone number

Name:

Address:

Tel:

I am registered with Dr

My endocrinologist

My pharmacist

Other members of my healthcare team

NOTES

SIMPLE GUIDE QUESTIONNAIRE

Dear reader,

We would love to know what you thought of this Simple Guide. Please take a few moments to fill out this short questionnaire and return it to us at the FREEPOST address below.

CSF Medical Communications Ltd
FREEPOST NAT5703
Witney
OX29 8BR

SO WHAT DID YOU THINK?

Which Simple Guide have you just read?

_____

Where did you buy it (store/town)?

_____

Who did you buy it for?

- [ ] Myself
- [ ] Patient
- [ ] Friend
- [ ] Other
- [ ] Relative

Where did you hear about the Simple Guides?

- [ ] They were recommended to me
- [ ] Stumbled across them
- [ ] Internet
- [ ] Other

Did it meet with your expectations?

- [ ] Exceeded
- [ ] Met most
- [ ] Met all
- [ ] Fell below

Was there anything you particularly liked?

_____

_____

_____

Was there anything we could have improved?

_____

_____

_____

WHO ARE YOU?

Name: _____

Address: _____

_____

_____

Tel: _____

Email: _____

How old are you?

☐ Under 25   ☐ 25–34   ☐ 35–44
☐ 45–54   ☐ 55–64   ☐ 65+

Are you...   ☐ Male   ☐ Female

Do you suffer from a long-term medical condition? If so, please specify.

_____

WHAT NEXT?

What other topics would you like to see covered in future Simple Guides?

Thanks,
     the Simple Guides team